CREATIVE CARE

CREATIVE CARE

A Revolutionary Approach to Dementia and Elder Care

ANNE BASTING

HarperOne
An Imprint of HarperCollinsPublishers

HarperOne

FIRST EDITION

Designed by Janet Evans-Scanlon

Illustrations by Violeta Noy

Library of Congress Cataloging-in-Publication Data

Names: Basting, Anne Davis, 1965- author.
Title: Creative care : a revolutionary approach to dementia and elder care / Anne Basting.
Description: First edition. | New York, NY : HarperOne, [2020]
Identifiers: LCCN 2019030876 (print) | LCCN 2019030877 (ebook) | ISBN 9780062906175 (hardcover) | ISBN 9780062906786 | ISBN 9780062992963 | ISBN 9780062906199 (ebook)
Subjects: LCSH: Dementia—Treatment. | Dementia—Patients—Care. | Older people—Mental health service. | Memory disorders in old age.
Classification: LCC RC521 .B3755 2020 (print) | LCC RC521 (ebook) | DDC 616.8/31—dc23
LC record available at https://lccn.loc.gov/2019030876
LC ebook record available at https://lccn.loc.gov/2019030877

20 21 22 23 24 LSC 10 9 8 7 6 5 4 3 2 1

Dedicated to the generations that wrap around me, my grandparents (Alice, Alice, Abe, and Arthur), parents (Tom and Sally), and my husband and boys (Brad, Ben, and Will). Let's laugh all the way through.

CONTENTS

PART THREE

Changing Care Through Creativity

PART ONE

Finding Creative Care

CHAPTER 1

In Which Ruth Teaches Me What Joy Looks Like

It was opening day. Spirits were incredibly high. I had walked into Morgantown Care and Rehabilitation in Morgantown, Kentucky, that Saturday morning to a chorus of exuberant greetings, not what you'd usually expect at a nursing home. Now it was just about 2 p.m.—showtime. After two weeks of rehearsal and a year of planning, the elders, local actors, volunteers, and staff were about to perform their version of *Peter Pan*—one in which Wendy is in hospice care in her final phase of growing up. And the audience, rather than clapping to prove their belief in fairies, would meet the extended hand of an elder to prove that they believed—in one another. There would be song and dance, there would be a giant crocodile, pirates, and of course flying. These residents, several of whom had not been out of their rooms for months, were about to welcome an audience to see them and their nursing home in a completely new light. They were inviting the audience to see beauty and meaning in a place where most people see only overwhelming loss.

Ruth had been at every rehearsal. If I had to guess, I would say Ruth was in her late eighties, with a bob of gray hair framing her face. Riding a wheelchair, she was one of the dozen elders dancing in the finale to Frank Sinatra singing "Fly Me to the Moon." As Shirley, a resident who had been the activity director in this very nursing home for forty years, offered a blessing on the performance, and the stage manager called out, "Places!" Ruth's care partner wheeled her out onto the home's front patio for the pre-show. The wind carried a chill, but every elder in the dance chorus insisted on going outside to greet the audience and listen to the live music. I looked around at the faces. Every one of them was wide-eyed and wonder-filled. Except Ruth. She was crying. Her eyes were bright, but tears rolled down her cheeks. Her mouth was twisted into a half-smile, half-grimace. I went to her straight away, kneeling down in front of her and taking her hands. "Ruth!" I whispered. "Are you okay?"

She nodded eagerly.

"Are they happy tears?" I asked.

"Oh, yes," she said with a laugh. "Happy, happy tears."

"Happy tears"—there's no better phrase to capture a feeling of joy in a time of tremendous challenge, such as when we create and experience poignant beauty in, say, a time of dementia, or a time of profound physical changes, or a time of powerfully missing people who have gone on before you or who are too far away or too busy to visit. In my twenty-five years of bringing the arts to people in late life, almost no one believes me when I first suggest it is possible to feel joy in these moments. Or that joy and meaning can coexist in some of the hardest times of our lives, if we are lucky enough to live that long. The power of being invited into creating meaning, of working together to create art that has a lasting legacy, is an elusive thing to describe. But when people feel it, they understand it deeply. I'm fairly confident that in the beginning of their training, the staff at the nursing home in Morgantown didn't believe in that power. Nor did the elders, or their families. But after the show, they sure believed—in themselves, in one another, and in the power of the shared creative experience.

I didn't always believe either. I didn't even know it was a thing that could be believed in. My journey toward the performance of *Wendy's Neverland* in a nursing home in Morgantown was a long, slow discovery for me, a gradual accumulation of experiences rather than a lightning strike. I continue to learn every day, especially now, as the landscape of time shifts under my own feet, bringing changes to my own family. It is my hope that the stories I've gathered here, stories of how I learned to apply the insights from theater and creativity studies to the world of elder care and memory loss, stories of bringing joy and connection to those who thought these possibilities were gone, stories from my many encounters with elders and care partners, offer readers a similar journey toward discovery—a journey toward believing that beauty, growth, learning, and joy are all possible in moments that most people assume to be overwhelmed only by loss and sorrow. My hope is that by reading this book you can follow in my footsteps and transform your relationships with people experiencing dementia and other challenges that can accompany aging.

There's an urgency to my hope of course. At this point, nearly everyone knows someone who is experiencing symptoms of physical and cognitive changes that can come with age. Some are mild, not much more than a nuisance and a topic for bonding laughter at dinner parties. Some progress cruelly in ways that bring dramatic changes to every aspect of our lives.

This person might be your neighbor. He might pause when he sees you, squinting to try to recall your name, then turning and hurrying back to close the door before you have a chance to offer your usual warm greeting. This person might be your wife of many, many years—an unfamiliar knot of worry growing behind her brows, a slight, haunting distance when your eyes meet. This person might be your father, in your mind always regal and confident, now hesitant and uncharacteristically cautious.

With the numbers as they are now, with successes in public health increasing life expectancy across the world, we are in a new era of adjusting to the realities of living into late life and the range of changes that might bring—whether physical or emotional. How will we navigate them? As sons and daughters? As spouses? As neighbors? How will we navigate these changes as communities? As cultures? As a species?

This has, of course, also been a personal journey. Mine has been long and slow, a million steps toward understanding the ideas at the root of "creative care." Just as I set out as a young scholar and artist, bucking stigma and market forces to focus my attention on aging and dementia, whole fields began to form around me. I had the dumb luck of falling into an idea whose time had come. In the beginning, I didn't know what a boomer was. But they were already starting to rattle the bars of the cage that kept stereotypes of aging in place. The academic field of age studies was already starting to form in the humanities as I started my dissertation. Disability studies came into its own and now has departments and centers, majors and minors across the world. Creative aging formed as a field, with nonprofit arts companies popping up from San Francisco to London. It was built by pioneers like Pam Schweitzer, Gene Cohen, Susan Perlstein, Stuart Kandell, and Ann McDonough, to name just a few, whom I have had the great fortune to know and call colleagues and friends.

I first stepped into this work in my twenties. Inevitably, this meant that when I told people that I worked with people with dementia using the arts, brows would furrow and eyes would narrow. The thought bubble above their heads—with the words sometimes also spoken aloud, sometimes not—asked, "Why would you want to do *that*?" and then "Do you have someone in your family with dementia?" The answer was too complicated for passing conversations. My response was usually, "No, not really." That was never satisfying to anyone. Brows furrowed more deeply. I was an aberration. Aging and dementia are depressing, those brows said. No one *really* wants to think about it, let alone a young woman in her twenties with light and hope leaking from every pore.

In my thirties and on through my forties, I continued to think and write about aging, and how the arts could both reshape how people think about aging and foster growth and meaning in late life. I followed in the footsteps of community-engaged artists working in fields of criminal justice, housing and homelessness, environmental justice, and education. Many of the stories in this book are from that period of creative experimentation, when I began to step away from traditional scholarship of my earlier books and more toward art-making with elders who became collaborators and friends. They generously opened themselves to risk and growth in the creative process and shared with me their stories of pushing through challenges like failing memories, physical frailty, and crises of confidence to make something beautiful, together.

Then, after more than twenty years in the field, just as I crested my fifties, dementia touched my inner sphere. The moment of realization was deceptively simple. I was washing dishes at my parents' cabin in their beloved north woods. It was here that they created rituals for me and my siblings and then for our children over the past twenty-five years: Announcing all arrivals of hummingbirds and pileated woodpeckers. Dock-sitting at sunset. Trying to catch that enormous (mythic) walleye. Walking the overgrown path to the river under bowering poplar trees.

We had just finished one of the handful of cabin meals—burgers and brats on the grill, which Dad was scrubbing while Mom and I restored order to the tiny kitchen. As I washed and piled various pots and bowls into the drying rack, Mom toweled them off and put them away—a whirling dance that folded time over on itself, year after year, summer after summer, Fourth of July after Fourth of July.

Then she stopped. She held up the salad bowl and paused.

"Where does this go?"

It was just a question. No trace of worry or confusion. No thought that this should be something she should know.

But for me, it was a collision of twenty-five of years studying and working with people with dementia—other people's parents and friends, spouses and siblings—and the emotional entanglements of my own life. And I knew what her question meant. It meant that when Mom looked at this object, it was suddenly and surprisingly foreign to her. She reached for the map of the kitchen in her mind, and it was gone. Object. Map. The connection was lost. Executive function. Conceptual thinking. A sign.

How to answer her? I had so many answers for the people who asked me questions in workshops and after keynote speeches. Or for the staff who asked me questions during demonstration sessions. But how to answer now?

"I think it goes up here," I said, "but if you can't find it later, just ask me and I'll remind you where we decided to put it."

It's okay. I'm here. It'll be okay. I will remember.

My mother and my grandmother were a bit like oil and water. But Mom did inherit Grandma's obsession with family stories and making sure future generations knew not just who came before them, but also stories that captured the nuances of their personalities, their talents and dreams, their tragic flaws. I must have six books that my mother has created over the years, at first hand-typed and copied, then painstakingly laid out in clumsy home publishing programs, photos cut and copied and pasted onto paper and run through the copier. Later the books were scanned and cut and pasted with digital magic. I paged through them after I first unwrapped them, then stored them—somewhere.

"Have you even read them?" she asked me once. I tried to explain that I saw them as reference books—something you refer to, but not something you sit down with and really read. She wasn't buying it. But that wasn't stopping her from writing more. One summer she signed up for a writing retreat held at a nearby college. It was for people writing fiction. She submitted her family stories anyway, got in, and used the time to gather together and write about all the letters she had written to a childhood mentor who had generously kept and given them all back to her as a chronicle of her emerging adulthood. "Who am I?" she seemed to be asking. "Who is this person in the letters?"

But now, in the kitchen, on a warm July night, Mom stopped and paused again. This time she stared at the family pasta bowl as though she had never before contemplated such a silly object. This object that we have used, washed, and put away a thousand times.

"Where does *this* go?" She sounded bemused.

I had been passive, even a little dismissive about Mom's obsession with family memories. I found her drive to write and pass them down—to labor through both the old-school scissors and paste and the learning of new software programs in her seventies—charming.

"Let's try up here. I think I remember seeing it up here," I said.

In that moment, as I nested the pasta bowl back into the stack of bowls where it had lived so efficiently for twenty-five years, the shift began. I could see that my sister and brother and I would be the keepers of those stories now, and I was washed by a wave of gratitude for her labor. For the paste. The scissors. The stories. The love that made them stick.

It's okay. I'm here. It'll be okay. I will remember.

My labor is now bound in hers. Mom is navigating with determination diagnoses and everyday moments transformed by a changing brain. When she and Dad told me of the diagnosis, Mom kept laughing. "I kept thinking," she said with a rolling laugh, "if they test me for three hours, there must be something up there to test!" "It's good you can laugh, Mom," I said. "This scares a lot of people." She suddenly got quiet. "Oh, I've made a decision to laugh, honey," she said flatly. "All the way through this." Her strength inspires me to discover my own. I aim to understand what is happening through her stories as I gather my own—to relay the essence of the work I have lived and slowly learned from for the last several decades and to push myself to read its possibilities in both directions in my life. Forward, to my mother, my father, my own aging. Back toward my younger students, who I know still get the furrowed brow in response when they tell people they work in aging; and toward my children, who are watching and navigating the changes in their grandparents and, in turn, their own parents.

Although dementia is never a welcome addition to one's life, it is giving me a chance to live my work with thickened emotions. Dementia has tested and will continue to test my ability to embrace the power and joy of the creative process overlaid with the losses that our lives inevitably present us simply as a result of staying alive over time. Dementia brings me and my family to that deepest place of meaning, where our human frailty and our unique human capacity to imagine entwine. Where we can experience breathtaking beauty and heart-wrenching sorrow simultaneously. Dementia brings us to creative care.

This book is for all of us navigating the terrain of dementia or late life's myriad challenges, whether you've chosen to work in the field of care or whether time and chance are bringing things like loneliness, confusion, and fear to people you love—or to you yourself. It is difficult terrain. No one can be expected to walk sure-footed amid such physical, emotional, and financial chasms. But the terrain is not *only* difficult. The elements of creative care I share here can embolden our steps with the hope and confidence that we *can* connect to the people we fear are lost to us, that we *can* create and experience meaning and joy along the way. The creative care approach invites us to shift away from the temptation to focus so heavily on losses and instead train our eyes and hearts on the strengths that remain. When we do, we can build on those strengths and make something new, together. Creating and opening shared moments of meaning-making is a power that we all have. But after a century of the arts being professionalized, we need assurance to tap into our innate skills of imagination. Learning to invite someone into imagination has the power to transform our relationships. It also has the power to change the way we think about aging and late life and the very systems we've built to control and support late life. The steps I outline and the stories I have gathered here are reminders that we all have that power inside us.

The stories in this book are not melodramas, in which the mustache gives away the bad guy and the endings are neatly tied. These are real-life stories, in which people are scared of the unknown, hold too tightly to old hurts, and are sad to lose people they love or to see them in pain. Yet these are also stories in which people open themselves to nearly overwhelming experiences of beauty and joy in the midst of loss. This new landscape can be nourished by many, many happy tears.

CHAPTER 2

The Upside of Having No Friends

Where did my journey toward caring for those with dementia using the imaginative arts start, what I have come to call "creative care"? I figured out the "creative" part long before the "care" part. As a quiet middle child, I would disappear into multiverses of imagination. As best I can remember, the habit started with bark, moss, and twigs that I would shape into little natural wonderlands of ground, grass, and trees. Sometimes, I admit, my wonderland might have included googly eyes. These weren't works of art by any means. But playing with scale, I was making malleable worlds that I could enchant. And that my tiny fingers could control. The habit extended to drawing too. I tended toward obsessive pencil drawings. Endless cross-hatching filled me with a joy that only a psychologist might explain. But I was also the kid who toted around an old typewriter box that I called my "briefcase" filled with old forms that I relished filling out—which probably explains quite a bit. Gradually, my arts habit grew to using words. My father always had a boundless vocabulary that I, his little mynah bird, would echo to build myself more multiverses. In sixth grade I remember the intoxicating feeling of falling into worlds peopled with characters that I had created. I named them, shaped their personalities, decided what they would wear, how they would talk and see the world. This seemed a miracle to me—surely other people must know about this power?

Things accelerated in middle school, when, thanks to some mundane mean-girl antics, I found myself with just one friend for nearly three years. That was an awful lot of pressure on that one friend, so I often relieved her and spent time alone. My mom was a champ. With kids of my own now, I realize how hard it was on her to watch me experience that and resist simply telling me, "Snap out of it!" or "It'll pass," neither of which makes sense to a middle schooler for whom time has no meaning and every emotion is a tsunami. Instead, she put me in art classes with a local painter. Her class of middle-aged stay-at-home moms, retirees, and professionals welcomed a taciturn thirteen-year-old with open arms. Together we drew landscapes, still lifes, and portraits. We fell into the worlds we were shaping with charcoal, ink, and paint, forgetting for a delicious hour or so the realm outside the art-room doors.

By the time my old friends came up to my locker in ninth grade to offer an olive branch (I genuinely thought they were going to fight me at first), I was probably beyond repair. I was used to hanging out with adults with settled lives. Conversations with my peers baffled me. Pencils, pens, and color became my way of reconciling the worlds I lived between. And they have been ever since.

Lessons from My Wordless Grandmother

The first question people ask me when I explain the work I do is, "Were you close with your grandmother?"—followed by, "Did someone in your family have dementia?" That scenario would make the most sense, of course, but it wasn't true, at least not at the start. As I said before, my journey has been long and slow. I was friendly with my grandmother. She was an adult, which meant I found her eminently more relatable than people my own age. But I only saw her a couple times a year. She was quite a character, though, and eventually we formed a strong bond. And there was indeed a moment after college when I went to visit her on my own, in which the worlds of care and creativity first collided for me.

It was thirty years ago now. I had no idea it was going to be a threshold moment—that years later I would be part of an international movement to transform long-term care. There was a whole lot I didn't know. I didn't know about the baby boom, or the demographic shifts that would create a new dynamic between young and old across the world. I didn't know about what it meant to a family to figure out how to pay for, or to provide themselves with, dignified elder care. I didn't know just how heavy a load it can be to carry memories for both yourself and someone who is in the midst of losing theirs. I didn't know how much I would come to love this work, even though it can be heavy—and really, really hard.

Back then, I was just visiting my Grandma Alice. I had driven three and a half hours up to northern Wisconsin to visit Alice in her new home, one built of cinder block and industrial cleanser. One that would be the last home of everyone who lived in it. The one-floor, prairie-esque building overlooked the farms and forests on the out-skirts of Shawano, which I had learned over the years of visiting my mother's family to pronounce "Shaw-no." Like an oxymoron in a warm southern drawl: Shaw. No. Like the building itself, which tried so hard to feel welcoming to those of us who dragged ourselves through the front door, and the feeling of panic that struck you the minute you stepped in: Shaw. Noooooooo.

My spirited grandmother had run out of options. She tormented the poor couple whom my uncles had arranged to live with her at home after her stroke. One too many nights of Grandma getting up in the dead of night and turning down the heat had sent them pack-ing. No replacements could be found.

It had been a remarkable run: Seven siblings on a Montana ranch. A one-way train ticket to Chicago at age eighteen. Night nurse su-pervisor at a prominent Chicago hospital. Swept away to Shawano by a country doctor from a family of country doctors. Four children. Twelve grandchildren. A ferocious will that couldn't stop the stroke from deadening her tongue. At age seventy-eight, this woman with stick-straight posture and a bossy streak, found herself unable to read, write, or get the last word—or any word at all.

Alice and I had grown fairly close over the years. Looking at pic-tures of her as a young woman on the ranch outside Bozeman, full chaps and a ten-gallon hat, I liked to imagine that I resembled her. Spending the occasional weekend with Grandma, we would watch news and classic movies on public television, talk current events, and exchange exercise tips. I also found it intriguing to bond with the woman who could drive my mother crazy. The only daughter with three brothers, Mom came to loggerheads with Grandma on a regu-lar basis. But I only rarely caught glimpses of that Alice. To me, she was strong-willed, smart, and adventuresome. It was an added bonus that she had a solid sense of style and was willing to share hand-me-downs. I built a quirky look from church rummage sales and Grandma's closet. I would not say that Alice was a warm and fuzzy grandmother type—or even that she was consistently nice. I still smarted from the time she taught me to ride horses at the family farm. I got settled into the saddle and looked to her for guidance. Instead, she hit the horse in the hindquarters, it reared up, and I fell hard in what I would like to remember as a humiliating pile of manure (but I can't verify that last detail). "Now get back on, and you'll be able to ride anything, anytime." She was right of course, but I didn't ride all that often. What I learned was how to handle her. I placated, cajoled, and pushed back with a glint in my eye. I loved the sharp edges of her brittle humor and her formidable strength, which even now eludes me. I loved her and the person I hoped I could become in her shadow. By the time I walked through the doors of the nursing home, she and I had shared more than a few moments of vulnerability and frank talk. When I graduated from college, she picked out a pearl lapel pin from a local jewelry store for me.

"Grandma, it's lovely, but I don't own a lapel," I tried to explain, "I don't know that I'd ever wear it."

"Well, what do you want?" I remember her asking, somewhat put out.

I told her I would love that old turquoise bracelet she got when she took a horse trip across the Navajo lands in the 1920s.

"That's too good for you!" she scoffed.

But by the end of the weekend, I drove away feeling the heavy weight of old turquoise embedded in melted silver dollars around my wrist, like one of Wonder Woman's magic cuffs.

Back at the nursing home, I made my way down the empty hallway to her room. I heard a soft, high-pitched, anonymous "help me." The voice, drifting into the empty hallway, repeated rhythmically, setting a heartbeat of the place.

Footstep, footstep. "Help me." Footstep, footstep. "Help me."

Grandma was in her room, and when she saw me (did she know I was coming?) her eyes, already enormous behind her thick glasses, widened. She was happy to see me. She motioned toward the door and to her wheelchair and I took my stance at the helm of the chair, following her crooked finger pointing the way to the sunny common room at the end of the hallway. There we sat, and there, with no words, she told me a story that would set the course for the next thirty years of my life.

Grandma had just three tools for communication. A single sound, which as best I can express it phonetically was something like "tsss tsss." She could shift its tone along a continuum from emphatic (you idiot!) to coaxing (oh, come now, you can do it—you're almost there). Second, she had that incredibly expressive index finger, bent with arthritis and pulsing with palsy, which seemed to point in two directions at once. It wasn't precise, but she could point in general directions and shake it with frustration. She was good at exasperation. Third, she had those enormous pale blue eyes that she could open and close for emphasis. Opening wider seemed to read, "Yes, yes!" Slowly closing was a sorrow that needed no translation.

"Help me," the voice echoed down the hallway.

In the sunny common room on the day of my visit, Grandma pointed out the window and opened her eyes wide. Clearly, I was supposed to say something.

"Outside?"

The crooked finger shook, and the "tsss tsss" scolded me. *You idiot.*

"Someone in Shawano?"

Clearly not.

"Someone beyond Shawano?"

Clearly yes.

"A relative?"

Yes.

Thirty minutes and about five hundred questions later, I arrived at the end. I was to drive to her house, look in the bottom drawer of her desk, and find an envelope with a return address that would tell me how I could be in touch with my mom's cousin who is a clinical psychologist—which is what Grandma had decided I should be. Enough with this arts stuff; I would help people. With a "tsss," a finger shake, and her haunting eyes, she managed to scold me, switch my vocational plans, and put me in touch with a relative I didn't know I had. It was exhausting and miraculous at the same time. With just those three tools she clawed her way out of her carapace. She made her will known. She showed me she knew me—knew something about me that I might not yet know about myself. She cared for me. Even if she was a little bossy.

But I had knowledge too. What Alice didn't know was that her house was being cleaned out by grieving and aggravated adult children. The house would be sold to pay for care. There was no envelope. There was no desk.

Help me, I thought.

I held her hands, looked her in the eyes, and told her I would ask Mom about it. I wheeled Alice back to her room. She didn't point the way.

My visit with Alice was short, but in that time I learned some profound things that would underscore every visit with each of the thousands of elders I've worked with since then:

* Everyone has stories inside them.
* Everyone has some kind of tool for expressing those stories.
* Everyone has barriers keeping their stories from coming out—some more than others.
* It is up to us to figure out how to invite the story out and how to listen it into existence.

After my experience with Alice, and over the many years of working with elders that would follow, I have come to see myself as a facilitator to the expression of stories. And I have also come to see, as I would later learn anthropologist Barbara Myerhoff had eloquently written, that stories are actually shaped in the relationship between teller and listener. I also learned, quite viscerally, that sorrow, loss, and growth, expression and learning, all coexist. "Help me" became my reminder. I never saw the woman whose plea set the refrain to my grandmother's nursing home, but I did wonder what other stories that woman might have if someone knew how to unlock them. What might "help me" come to express in its fullness?

I drove away from the nursing home, not knowing it would be the last time I would see Alice. I remember the time as sunset, but it probably wasn't. I drove to her house on the Wolf River, where I began the work my mother had charged me with: figure out which things of Grandma's I wanted to keep. What tangible reminders could possibly hold the memory of that feisty spirit? Or more practically, perhaps, which items could help me set up my apartment in graduate school where I would definitely not be studying clinical psychology, but rather pursuing a doctorate in theater that would later morph into a study of the performance of aging?

Now, with hindsight, I wonder whether the two paths of study were so different after all.

Much of my work after that moment with Alice has been to create tools that can bring people into deeper relationships with one another and with the current and future world around them through the medium of imagination and the creative arts. You certainly don't need to be a clinical psychologist or have a PhD in theater studies to invite someone to express themselves, to echo their responses, and to infuse those responses with value by sharing them with the broader world. This is what I have come to call creative care: a mutually nurturing and generative process for both teller and facilitator. This process helps people move through the barriers to connecting with elders (or anyone for that matter)—the fear, the guilt, the grief, to name just a few—and to feel confidence in people's creative capacity to facilitate and experience meaningful connection together. This process can bring us back to one another and teach us the power of the very human act of caring for one another.

In this first part I share my long, slow journey in discovering this revolutionary approach while also explaining the context for the current state of our care for those with dementia. Maybe others would have figured it out earlier, but it took an accumulation of experiences for me to arrive at creative care. I share stories of Grandma, of my unique journey as both an artist and a scholar. I share a story from another moment in a nursing home, this time not with my grand-mother, but several years and many miles away, with a half-dozen elders suffocating under the weight of sedation, isolation, and shrill alarm bells. And again, I was stunned to find that the simple power of imagination was enough to lift that weight and enable us to reach each other.

In the second part of the book, I focus more specifically on the elements of creative care and how they can help transform our relationships. Here is where you will receive concrete instructions for how you, too, can participate in this important work. Caring for a friend or family member, particularly in situations of dementia, is hard, hard work, both physically and emotionally. I use stories from over the years that bring moments of creative care out of conceptual descriptions and into real-life situations. I try to formalize the steps as much as possible to make it easy for everyone to try, even when energy and resilience are low. While the elements of creative care emerged through my work with people with dementia, these elements also have guided and improved my relationships in teaching, the workplace, and parenting. Creative care can enrich any of the relationships in our lives.

In the third part, I explore the promise of creative care to transform not just our relationships, but also our care systems. Here I share stories of bold, creative projects that push against the status quo of "activities" and low expectations for learning in late life. I start with the story of the Penelope project, which brought a professional theater company, university theater students, and the elders, families, and staff of an entire long-term-care community into collaboration to reinterpret Homer's *Odyssey* and stage an original play in the community itself. The lessons from Penelope ignited my curiosity about what else could be done to invite elders into meaning-making. I then share the story of the Islands of Milwaukee project, designed to engage elders living alone at home. One particular "artistic house call" that I made during that project became a powerful lesson in adjusting to temporal dissonance—also known more simply as slowing down. The magic of singing and exchanging stories with Bill never would have happened if I hadn't let time slip a bit—a lesson that could change how we understand and practice home care.

The third part of the book also features the story of a program called SAIR, or Student Artists in Residence, in which several student artists each year live in care settings in a mutual learning experience. I have learned so much from this program, through the students' reflections and realizations of just how segregated by age their worlds were, and through the gentle mentorship and creative risk-taking of their elder friends.

The Crossings project tells the story of how elders of all abilities can go way, way beyond bingo to be engaged in shaping the world around them. The Crossings was a street performance to teach drivers to see and stop for pedestrians in the hope of raising the street-crossing confidence of elders living near the intersections. I also share the story of the power of several choirs that are growing in popularity across the United States. Part 3 of the book ends with the story of my largest project yet, a reimagining of the story of Peter Pan in collaboration with the elders, staff, and families at twelve rural nursing homes across Kentucky. The "I Won't Grow Up" project, as we called it, culminated in spring 2019 with three original, professionally produced plays at three of those twelve nursing homes. It was there that Ruth (and I, and so many others) cried our happy tears.

What can we learn from these stories? In the end, I hope to point a way toward joy and meaning for the millions of families wrestling with frailty, isolation, and cognitive challenges in late life. This path can help us all approach our relationships with older people and build systems to support our own aging if we are not yet there. Drawing on the voices and experiences of the elders I've had the privilege to work with and learn from over the past thirty years, this book is part map, part manifesto to fuel larger-scale changes to our care systems and our cultural and educational systems that will enable creative care to flow through them like water, nourishing both listener and teller, carer and cared for, in a mutually meaningful shaping of the world.

But first, let's return to the lessons of my mythic, ornery, somewhat loving cowgirl grandmother.

What I Learned by Not Going to Grandma Alice's Funeral

I took my first step toward realizing elder care should look radically different from the way it usually does when I skipped my grandmother's funeral to watch a vaudeville-style performance by elder actors. This story took place in spring in Minneapolis, just a year after my visit with Alice in the nursing home. My mom was in town visiting me for her birthday, and I was hosting a brunch in her honor. We were just digging into the chocolate gâteau when the phone rang. Grandma Alice had died. Mom didn't say anything, but I could see the thought bubble rise above her head: "On my birthday. Classic."

The plans took shape over the next couple of hours. The funeral would fall on the same day that I had arranged interviews with a senior theater troupe as part of my dissertation research. I was set to travel to Brainerd, Minnesota, to see a performance of the Geritol Frolics and to talk with a handful of the hundred-plus-member troupe. It wasn't an easy ticket to get. The Frolics offered a biannual, professional-quality vaudeville-style review complete with more than twenty costume changes. Tickets regularly sold out in fifteen minutes. I had to compete with tour guides and activity directors from area care homes who bought tickets by the busload.

"Oh, for God's sake, go!" said my mom in her most matter-of-fact voice. "Your grandmother would roll over in her grave if she knew you were sacrificing your career for her funeral."

Even though that wasn't technically possible yet, my mom had a point. Still, funerals aren't really for the dead. I had to decide whether I could process Alice's death on my own. In my late twenties at the time, I had never been to a funeral before. A winter storm kept me from my grandfather's memorial a few years earlier. With hindsight, I would have rescheduled and relished the rare company of my cousins, aunts, and uncles, who rarely gathered again after Alice's passing. But at the moment, without any real sense of the ritual or the emotions funerals were meant to welcome and exorcise, I decided to keep the interview appointments.

I had been writing both fiction and nonfiction about older people since my undergraduate English adviser was kind enough to allow me to write a (rather bad) play for my senior thesis. The play—go figure!—was about a young man whose grandfather had lost the ability to speak, and the two of them invent a shared world together. When I started my master's degree in theater, I was in a program focused on representations of and by women. No one was writing about representations of older women. I saw a void and stepped into it. By the time I got to the dissertation, I was thrilled to have found the "senior theater movement," which was relatively new in the early 1990s. Across the United States, Canada, the United Kingdom, and continental Europe, groups of older people who yearned to perform were banding together. Some had harbored dreams of acting for decades, and retirement now freed them from their more practical careers. Others were professional actors tired of being sidelined by ageism.

Just a year earlier, in 1993, I thought I was the luckiest person in the world to be attending the first Senior Theater Festival, held in Las Vegas. Ten senior performing groups, from Fresno, California, to Baltimore, Maryland, were gathered to perform and learn from one another. At twenty-eight, I was one of the youngest attendees, one of the only playwrights, and one of the only academics. My unicorn status might have been odd to the elders gathered there, but not to me. I had spent weekends hanging out with my grandmother watching *Gigi* or *Doctor Zhivago*. On a monthlong class in Chicago, I hung out with my grandmother's best friend, Rose, drinking strawberry daiquiris at all the once and formerly hip restaurants. Walking into a conference session as the only person under age sixty was normal to me, even if the performances were not really my style of theater. I was more of a Samuel Beckett kind of person. I loved vivid, poetic plays rich in images that invoked new worlds. The majority of these showcase performances were vaudeville-style reviews sprinkled with favorite scenes from Broadway musicals. But style aside, there was no denying the exhilaration and pride emanating from the festival, and the Geritol Frolics' performance was the showstopper. *You're as Young as You Feel* was a three-hour review, a "side-splitting comedy and dance extravaganza" (as the promotional materials promised) replete with kicklines and tap routines. A woman sitting next to me, a performer for another troupe at the festival, leaned over to me during one of the many extravagant dance routines and whispered with concern, "We're supposed to follow that??"

In the spring of 1994, the Frolics were set to perform a new, slightly scaled-down review called *Memories of the Thirties*. It clocked in at just two hours with a cast of sixty people ranging in age from their early seventies to their early nineties. Several of the Frolics performers generously agreed to meet with me in a small conference room near the theater a few hours before the performance. So a week after my Grandma Alice had passed, rather than drive east to Shawano, I went north to Brainerd. Just two and a half hours north of Minneapolis, through Little Falls (home of Charles Lindbergh), and through a knotty emotional thicket of grief that I chose to ignore. I reminded myself multiple times—Mom said it was okay.

The performers wore their iconic Geritol Frolics red sweatshirts and they welcomed me with a warmth that put a crack in my veneer. First around the conference table were Leonard and Eleanor Bagne, who had been part of the original cast in 1986, part of the early vision of their beloved founding director, Bob Dryden. I didn't ask their ages, but the long-married couple matched my notion of what the vigorous late eighties might look like. Leonard and Eleanor had been drawn to Dryden's vision by his insistence that the Frolics commit themselves to professional-quality shows. This was a significant difference from the other senior theater work emerging at the time, which was based on reminiscence and therapy. The Frolics had rigorous rehearsal and production expectations. This wasn't, as Leonard put it, a "tin pan and kazoo type of thing, a kitchen utensil type of show."

The rewards of being involved with the Frolics were clear, but the demands were, too. I asked the Bagnes how long they thought they might stay in the cast. Leonard paused, then said quietly, "Every year we wonder which will be the last for us, because I think the nature of show business is that you need new faces and new talent and so on, and we probably can't contribute much anymore other than to be a body up there on the stage."

"Oh—but a body on stage can be so beautiful!" I wanted to say to them. In the theatrical world of Samuel Beckett, some characters simply opened and closed their mouths, and the impact was stunning. In my mind, thin, soft lines in the skin made the face so much more expressive. Older performers don't have to imitate younger ones to be a powerful presence on stage. I had seen an eighty-seven-year-old butoh dancer move so slowly he seemed to reveal the source of life itself. The Frolics sold out their shows in fifteen minutes. They complained that they couldn't go to the local diner anymore without being recognized. But the Frolics' notion of professional theater seemed to preclude bodies, eyes, ears, minds that couldn't withstand twenty-eight costume changes and bright lights. Helen Molin, whom I interviewed after the Bagnes, told me she had tripped on a riser on her way off stage last year, the lights blinding her: "I really hurt myself." I remembered Helen from the Vegas performance the year before. She walked on stage at her own pace, in her own time, tightly coiffed white hair, slightly bent at the shoulders, no more than five feet tall. She completely owned that room. When Helen found her spot, she looked out at the audience and delivered three groaner jokes with impeccable timing, and then walked back off stage. She was beautiful.

As best I can re-create it from notes and memory, Helen's interview captures the simple transformative power of performance for performers of any age.

"What did you do before the Frolics?" I asked her.

"I was a widow," she said matter-of-factly.

"What might be a typical day for a widow?" I asked.

"Well, we talk on the phone to our children who are far away. We go to church, and we watch television," she said, explaining it to me as if it were the most obvious thing in the world.

"And what do you do now that you are with the Frolics?" I asked.

"Well, now I am a comedian, so I read up on jokes. I ask people for jokes. I write them down. And I go to rehearsal." Her face brightened, her posture seemed to lift a bit, even though it seemed from her tone that rehearsal could also be a bit bothersome.

I asked Helen about the audition process.

"Well, I saw the notice in the paper. So I went down there. They asked me if I could sing. I said no. They asked me if I could dance. I said, 'Oh, no.' They asked me what I wanted to do for the audition. And I said 'It's your audition, you tell me!' So they gave me some jokes to read, and now I am a comedian."

Helen would have gotten along smashingly well with Grandma Alice.

Another interview, and another. In one, I share an observation that in the Senior Theater Festival, I notice that there weren't any wheelchairs or even canes used in the performances. What happens if someone has physical challenges? Or memory loss? Joan Witham, one of the Frolics dancers, assured me that the community is incredibly supportive: "They might not be on stage anymore, but we don't forget them."

Finally, it's my last interview before the performance. Until now, I have fought to keep the knot of grief in my stomach from crawling up into my throat. But it was a long drive to Brainerd, a long day, and my resistance is wearing down. As Frolics performer Ruth Meyer tells me about her husband's funeral a few years ago, and how the entire Frolics cast came to the ceremony, a sea of red Frolics sweatshirts surrounding the grave, the knot slips and rushes upward. I give up the fight. As Ruth consoles me, I wonder just how much I missed in the earlier interviews as I busied myself with my own denial of feelings of loss.

I find my way to my seat in the crowded theater. The place is abuzz. The tour buses have all unloaded, and older people from area care and senior centers are settling into their seats. I am thankful for an aisle seat toward the front, in case the knot slips again. Over the next two hours, one tap routine melts into the next. One of Helen's jokes is truly funny, but my face is frozen in the security of observation mode. There are nearly a hundred performers in the troupe. They have movement. They have voice. They have so much more than a twisted finger and a scolding "tss tss tss." There has to be something between the Rockette-style kicklines and completely disappearing from the stage. In theater and in life.

Clearly, this world of senior theater radically and positively transformed what the Frolickers imagined to be possible in their "old age." They went from accountant to choreographer, from wife and mother to tap dancer, from widow to comedian. Becoming performers in late life enabled them literally to take on new roles, to learn and to grow. The performers developed intensely supportive social networks, something research tells us is crucial to our physical and psychological well-being. These performers went from feeling invisible in their communities to being recognized on the street or at the local diner.

But did performance, a memory-based art that demanded so much from actors, preclude the participation of older people with physical or cognitive challenges? Did this world I had committed myself to with months of dissertation research have a place for my own grandmother? Or for her best friend and now my dear friend, Rose, with whom I'd shared so many strawberry daiquiris and late-night conversations? Rose, who the last time I visited her apartment lay stiff and tightly curled in a bed with metal railings?

I would spend the next two years trying to find out whether the transformative power of theater could be put in a jar and opened in cinder block nursing homes or in lonely rooms of frail and isolated elders avoiding nursing homes.

Gifts from the Worst Place
You Can Imagine

"I don't want to go," I say flatly on the phone to Brad, my boyfriend, who would later become my husband. He calmly reminds me that I said the exact same thing last week.

"I still don't want to go," I say.

But somehow I find myself driving west and pulling into the parking lot of the Marian Franciscan Center, a four-story nursing home on a busy thoroughfare in the western suburbs of Milwaukee. It is a nondescript, pale beige building with maroon trim. There's really nothing about it that makes you want to stop, and nothing much to look out the windows at when you are inside either.

Sitting in the car, I take a deep breath, willing myself to gain the momentum to cross the threshold of the sliding-glass doors.

I was in Milwaukee for a yearlong postdoctoral fellowship while I turned my dissertation into a book. It was a blessed existence for a recent graduate. My younger sister happened to be living in Milwaukee, too, and was looking for a roommate. Together we found a beautiful duplex just a few blocks down from the university, where I had an office on the ninth floor with a view of Lake Michigan. Our father had grown up in Milwaukee, and my sister and I spent our childhoods visiting our grandparents in their little bungalow on the south side of town. But both our grandparents were gone now, and Dad was an only child. So we were getting to know the city on our own. By chance, my father's cousin, whom we'd never met before, called to welcome us to town. I asked her what she did for work, and she said she was an activity professional at a local nursing home.

Bingo.

I had been haunted by the absence of disability in the senior theater movement. It was so clear that performance, taking on a new role in late life, could change the way people understood their own aging. Performance could change the way communities understood the older people in their midst. But in the two years I had been watching plays in the senior theater movement, I had seen exactly one person using a cane, and no one in a wheelchair. I wanted to see if theater could be as transformative for people with serious cognitive and physical disabilities.

So when my dad's cousin Bernadine, who happened to work in a nursing home, invited me to volunteer at the Marian Franciscan Center, I took her up on the offer. It wasn't easy. The place has changed considerably over the past twenty-five years, but as it was back then, if you closed your eyes and imagined your worst nightmare of a nursing home, you would have a solid mental picture of the Marian Franciscan Center. I'm sure that my recollections are colored by time and crystallized by emotion. But I vividly remember that as the sliding-glass doors opened, I had to inhale and swallow my breath, willing myself through an invisible curtain of the pungent smell of urine. I breathed through my mouth as I walked the long hallway to the stairs. I'd head up two flights to the third floor and into the chaotic common room of the locked dementia unit. The first thing I noticed was the sound. The television was blaring *Wheel of Fortune*, but no one was watching. The elders were sitting slumped in wheelchairs, four to a table, curved like capital Cs, heads down, spirits broken. The piercing "beep beep beep" of an alarm set off by one of the electronic bracelets signaled that one of the residents had tried to go through a door they shouldn't have—*probably to get away from the sound*, I thought. The staff seemed to have become inured to the alarm. Some days, the beeping never seemed to stop the whole time I was there. To add to the cacophony, a group of nuns gathered in wheelchairs in a corner of the room were listening to Mass on transistor radios at full blast. It was nearly impossible for me to think straight. I couldn't imagine what it felt like for someone with dementia. When I look back at the setting in my mind, I see a room of about twenty souls, eyes closed, grimacing with the effort to shut out the world. I don't remember seeing a staff member in that dayroom after my very first visit. This is the collective nightmare that fuels countless declarations and much pleading: *Never put me in a nursing home.*

It was in this setting that I had been volunteering, once a week for six weeks, when I called my boyfriend, Brad, to find that extra bit of courage to keep going. Before embarking on my volunteering, I had done copious research, juggling various combinations of search words: "Alzheimer's," "dementia," "arts," "theater," and "activities." There wasn't much out there. In 1995, the prevailing wisdom about dementia was to supply answers for people, filling in their blanks, orienting them to the day, the time, the season, the president. Orientation and reminiscence were the dominant approaches for inviting elders of all abilities into conversation. But when memories and cognition were challenged, the books simply told you to "be flexible." In my research, I found Dr. Ann McDonough's dissertation from a few years earlier, which was about adapting to work with adults "creative drama" techniques that had been designed for children. McDonough was the host of the Senior Theater Festival, and the creator of the first degree in senior theater in the United States, at the University of Nevada, Las Vegas. I figured she of all people would know the path. So I studied her creative drama techniques, which were really just simple theater exercises that invited people to use their imaginations and share memories. I brought a few of these exercises with me each week to the Marian Franciscan Center.

One week I picked a group of elders gathered around one of the tables and invited them to be trees.

"Can you be a tree?"

Nothing.

"How might you show me you are a tree?" I asked, with an encouraging smile.

Nothing.

I modeled a tree: arms up, fingers out. Perhaps if I made myself ridiculous, they'd laugh?

One woman, who had looked up with what I remember as a gaze of pity for me, was kind enough to copy me: arms lifted slightly, hands open.

"Great! That's good! Now what if you were a willow tree?"

Nothing.

"How might you be a willow tree?"

Nothing.

I modeled a willow tree, drooping my arms and fingers; and, bless her heart, she copied me again. I tried a wide variety of trees, bushes, and flowers. I tried windy days. I tried imagining rain. I asked for stories about trees, flowers, nature of any kind. Anything: sun, wind . . . No one initiated a response. Clearly, this wasn't working. Could they hear me? Could they comprehend my questions? Was I asking them to take too many cognitive steps? Was I giving them enough time? Was the dayroom just too chaotic? Were they simply too pharmaceutically restrained with layers of medications? Was I just being too ridiculous?

Week after week, I tried: Sensory questions. Questions about holidays. About children. Family. Vacations. Pets. I tried gentle movement. Inviting people to follow me. I went back through reminiscence guides. I poured over the creative drama exercises. Nothing seemed to work. I started to dread each week.

"I don't want to go," I'd say to Brad on the phone in the car.

"You said that last week, and then you were happy you went."

Was I? For six weeks, I seemed to be proving that the benefit of performance was for the well. Was there any way to invite these elders out of their pharmaceutically induced haze and into the world again? Out of this strange state of group solitary confinement and into meaningful connection with themselves and each other? I didn't have a social work degree. I didn't have the ability to bring them new pills. All I could bring with me was my hope, my sunny disposition, a total lack of information about their various diagnoses, some theater games, and a few art supplies.

These turn out to be exactly what is necessary.

In week seven of my volunteering mission, I again willed myself out of the car, through the urine curtain, up the stairs, and into the common room, bringing with me a big pad of paper, a few markers, and a picture torn out of a magazine—the iconic profile of the Marlboro Man under an enormous Stetson. Rather than ask them to remember stories of their own lives, which had inevitably led to blank stares, and which I gave up weeks ago, I asked them to *imagine*.

I introduce myself again to my four faithful elders, gathered around a table.

"This week," I say, "let's make up a story. Any story. You can say anything, and I'll write it down." Pointing to the picture of the Marlboro Man and feeling a little ridiculous, I ask, "What do you want to name him?"

One of them musters a soft "I don't know."

"I don't know either—you can just make it up," I reassure them.

Pause. I try again.

"What do you think is a good name for him? Any name you want."

One of the elders lifts his head slightly and says, "Fred."

A surge of joy rushes through me. This is the most response we've had in six weeks. This one-syllable name feels like a miracle.

"Fred who?"

"Fred Astaire," says another gentleman.

Someone chuckles. The miracle is doubled.

"Where do you want to say he is?" I ask.

There is a long, thoughtful moment of quiet.

"Oklahoma," someone says.

And a woman breaks the C curve, lifts her head, and softly and slowly sings, "Oklahoma, where the wind comes sweeping down the plain . . ."

We are all shocked. More heads lift.

"What is Oklahoma like?" *Am I pushing it?* I wonder.

"There are lots of skinny rivers. And skinny trees."

"Is he married?" I decide to roll with it as long as I can.

"Yes."

"To whom?" I ask.

"Gina Autry."

Ok. Now that's just plain funny. I can't stop smiling now, suspended in a moment that truly feels like a miracle. It's hard to catch my breath, I repeat what they had said so far to make sure they stay close to the heart of the story they are creating.

"So here we have Fred Astaire," I say, "he is married to Gina Autry, they live in Oklahoma—" (we take a moment to sing "Oklahoma" again) "where there are lots of skinny rivers and skinny trees."

Eventually, between my questions and their responses, we create a world in which Fred and Gina work in the rodeo. He does calf-roping and she does barrel-riding. They can't be in the same event, because she is better than he is. They don't have any kids; they don't have time. They tend black-and-white cows who say, "Hi, Pat." They have three dogs, Bozo, Sandy, and ABCDEFG. They will have a big Christmas dinner on a white lace tablecloth with candles. They will eat goose.

The story is funny, thoughtful, and peppered with what I'm sure are details drawn from real life, along with their playful imaginations and the residue of whatever disease is snarling their synapses. The common room and its chaos melt away. The storytellers and I are looking at one another, eyes shining. Then we notice that there are people standing around us. They appear to be staff. Their eyes are shining too. They look like they might be—what—jealous? Clearly, they want to play, too. I thank everyone profusely. It's incredible how hard the elders worked for nearly forty-five minutes. They answered every one of my silly questions. They came out and played, with me and with one another. It was a gift.

The session is over.

I don't want to go.

I don't want to break the spell. I'm afraid that if I leave that circle, it might never happen again, that we'll go back to being capital Cs, shutting out the world and staring at our laps. But I do; I have to. Visits end. The clock of the outside world keeps ticking.

I went back for six more weeks, until the end of my fellowship. Every week I repeated the same approach. I introduced myself. I brought a new image I had found on a greeting card or torn from a magazine and had copied so it was large enough for the elders to hold onto. I asked open-ended questions that invited any response they could make, and I repeated whatever answers they gave, whether they were sounds, movements, words I recognized, or words I didn't. I fell deep into the rhythms of improvisation and emerged each week with stories full of hopes, regrets, wicked humor, gentle teasing, longing, deep sorrow, and settled satisfaction. There were songs and stunning, accidental poetry that lifted all of us.

Now, with twenty-some years of hindsight, I can report that the magic came back every single time I tried this approach. In nursing homes. In senior centers. At kitchen tables. In lobbies of senior apartment buildings. The magic comes back for the thousands of people across the world whom we have trained through TimeSlips, a nonprofit organization I founded to study and share this approach. This simple shift, from an emphasis on memory toward the freedom of imagination, opens up meaning-making to those who thought it was beyond their reach. Grandma Alice taught me that everyone has a story. The elders at the Marian Franciscan Center taught me how to invite it, affirm it, echo it, build it, and celebrate it. That is the core of creative care.

PART TWO

Defining Creative Care

CHAPTER 3

When Opposites Come Together

I am often surprised that the idea of combining creativity and care is a new one. For me, the yearning to unite the concepts stemmed from my desire to bring together the two fields I had straddled for so many years. There was the world of the arts and its long hard slog of practice and honing technique in the hope of making something truly beautiful and the dream that people will recognize and be transported by that beauty. And there was the world of elder care, where so many full-hearted and well-intended (and a few not so well-intended) people fight denial, stigma, physically and emotionally demanding work, lack of funding, and intense regulations to carefully tend and mend the bodies and spirits of older people so that they might flourish in their final years. I had been working to bring these two worlds together my entire career. But suddenly, when I saw these two words, "creative" and "care," together, with no other words between them, they seemed foreign. What did this hybrid term even mean? Did I really know what the words meant separately?

The more I looked at the newly joined term, the more I could feel the tension between the words and the vibration of the potential born of this union. To understand the term more fully and, most important, to be able to explain it to others, I needed to refresh my understanding of each term individually. I started with "creativity."

What Is Creativity?

While it has been part of my life for as long as I can remember, it turns out that creativity is going through a moment in the spotlight. Creativity is cool. Or it was cool ten minutes ago, anyway. Studies on and about creativity have surged in the past several decades. I was a little surprised to find that there are now degrees in creative studies and that multiple academic journals are publishing research on how to be more creative in a variety of settings, from artist studios to corporate boardrooms. Some scientists are studying the neurobiology of creativity with magnetic resonance imaging (MRI) technology, while others are observing the conditions in which workers become more creative or researching which personality traits might be unique to highly creative people. No matter how many articles I read, I found consistency in how the term was applied. "Creativity" is used to identify and describe people, processes, and products. Creativity is considered to be a uniquely human characteristic, setting us apart from animals and machines.[1]

When I was first developing a training course in the improvisational storytelling technique, I leaned on Dr. Gene Cohen's definition of creativity from his book *The Creative Age*, one that he had in turn drawn from Rollo May and Mihaly Csikszentmihalyi: creativity is something new added to the world that has value. But that was way back in 2001. Was that still how this new surge of scholars in creativity studies defined it? I dove back into the research and found that while definitions were multiple and somewhat varied, in the end they nearly all settled on those same two basic points. Creativity is a process that (1) generates something novel or new that (2) has value.[2] I had always found a simple beauty in this definition—that it does not say who considers it new or valuable. The way that I adapt a recipe when I discover that the sour cream in the fridge has gone fuzzy is new and valuable to me (and to my kids who greedily devour the banana bread made with yogurt). Deafening cheers at the end of a concert reveal a different level of value—one conveyed by concert venues, huge audiences, and cultural critics. In the literature on creativity, you'll find these two levels are commonly referred to as "little c" or private creativity, and "Big C" or public creativity, respectively.[3]

I am a firm believer that "little c" creativity permeates the lives of all human beings, no matter how many times they might have been told that they are not creative. Whenever a person faces an unexpected obstacle, finding the way through (around, under, or over) a given challenge demands a novel solution and an adaptation in the person's routine. From coping with inconsolable toddlers in grocery store lines to dealing with co-workers who pick the day of an important presentation to get sick or stubborn, finding one's way in a new situation will yield new solutions that are valuable—especially to the people in line behind that toddler and to the boss counting on that presentation to generate a sale. Aging itself, living into a new day that presents new situations—some more challenging than others—invites us to exercise creativity with every breath.

When I introduce the concept of "little c" creativity in training workshops, I ask people to make a list of all the ways that they express creativity in their lives. Even for those who are adamant that they are not creative, somehow a list magically emerges: Gardening. Cooking. Figuring out the best route to drive in busy traffic. Handling conflicts at work. Giving the perfect gift. Decorating the house. Accessorizing an outfit. Picking out an outfit for a given occasion. Writing letters. Making ends meet. Parenting a challenging child. Keeping a relationship strong over time. And on top of those everyday forms of creativity, one can toss in the more traditional kinds of creativity, such as drawing, painting, photography, singing, playing an instrument, dancing, and writing poetry. Every mode we have to express ourselves can be used to express creativity.

The process of creating something new that has value demands a certain flexibility. One recognizes patterns, generates multiple possible solutions to the challenge (also known as *divergent thinking*), and breaks or stretches the rules or routines that guide a given practice.

In low-stakes situations, this process might also be called "play." As the pediatrician and psychoanalyst Donald Winnicott suggests, "In playing, and perhaps only in playing, the child or adult is free to be creative."[4] In play we can experiment with countless options and imagine alternative scenarios—also known as "make-believe." But for some people and in some cultures, play is strictly the terrain of the children. I have run into the wall of this view several times, usually in the form of an icy stare from an adult child standing guard over the dignity of his or her father. "My father would never do that" is the wall that comes down. Unfortunately, until now, the vast majority of the research on the benefits of play for learning and emotional well-being reinforces this notion, because this research largely focuses on children. But adults are certainly capable of and can benefit tremendously from play that is age-appropriate as well.[5]

My deep dive into the research on creativity confirmed my understanding that it is an essential part of human well-being. These ideas go way back. In Maslow's famous model of the hierarchy of human needs from 1943, he positions creativity as one of the paths that can lead to self-fulfillment.[6] Viktor Frankl, writing after his experience in Nazi death camps, saw the power of creating things as one of just three paths to a meaningful life.[7] In the field of positive psychology, creativity is seen as leading to well-being by helping us articulate a story about who we are (coherence); exercising a purpose; and demonstrating the significance or value of our lives. Creativity can also help us build a legacy, something that can live beyond us and that can reduce the stress, anxiety, or at the very least the unsettledness we can feel when we face mortality.

Creativity can also supply us with "peak" or "optimal" experiences.[8] One such peak experience has been called "flow," or the feeling of being so swept away in the creative process that one loses sense of time and place.[9] When I read about flow and the power of creativity to crowd out our everyday worries or pains, I am reminded of a story from the Penelope project, in which I worked with a team of artists, students, staff, and elders at a long-term-care community to reimagine Homer's *Odyssey* from the perspective of Penelope. Barbara, who lived in the nursing home, participated in every workshop she could. She pushed through her pain to create music, dance, write stories, and make weavings. One day when we were rehearsing for the play that emerged from the project, a nurse tracked her down in the hallway to deliver her medicine. "Barbara, I have your pain meds." Barbara waived her off. "I don't need them now," she said. A friend of mine who was on staff witnessed the moment and told me about it later, saying, "I think that's what this project was all about."[10]

Yet for all its benefits, creativity, like play, was long assumed to be the purview of the young. Gene D. Cohen's *The Creative Age* was pivotal in lifting the barrier separating creativity and late life. In this book Cohen eloquently advocates for seeing late life as a time when creativity can flower. "Creativity," he writes, "is a powerful inner resource that is not only possible in later life, but common."[11] I was one of the many lucky artists and scholars to know Dr. Cohen and counted both him and his wife, Wendy, as among my inspirations and friends. His presentations embodied play and imagination. With a sparkle in his eye and an umbrella covered in painted clouds above his head, for years Cohen pushed against this stubborn stereotype— that aging somehow meant increasing rigidity and loss of imagination. He cited research in brain plasticity and stories from both his practice and the art world to change hearts and minds. Besides the grin that would widen across his face when he showed a slide filled with chocolate ("Creativity is chocolate for the brain"), his favorite story was about Georgia O'Keeffe. In her later years, O'Keeffe overcame a lifelong fear of flying. The result was the magnificent series of paintings, *Sky Above Clouds*, and the inspiration for Cohen's umbrella. For Cohen, rising above the turbulence of fears and losses opened a whole new world of opportunities for growth.[12]

Clearly, creativity is good for us at any age, and research is only continuing to prove this. The aspect of Western notions about creativity that has always made me uncomfortable, however, is the mythology of the solo artist or creative genius. Cohen included a short chapter in *The Creative Age* on creativity in the context of relationships. But this perspective is surprisingly rare. For too long, creativity studies have focused on creativity solely as an individual process. Western cultures love to make heroes (tragic, comic, or otherwise) of the creative genius, working alone on an idea, laboring for years against the grain of prevailing thought until one day, ideally before the genius's death, his or her ideas are recognized as a breakthrough. A story that commonly follows the one of the unexpected solo genius, however, is the one about the overlooked collaborators who never got the credit they deserved. Yet our ideas about and research on creativity have been slow to expand beyond the individual. I was heartened to find that in the past decade, creativity scholars have started to expand their view—to move out of the studio or lab, and into dynamic relationships between people, in which ideas bounce back and forth and evolve into new and valuable thinking or creative artifacts. As one scholar of creativity reminds us, "No one ever invented the wheel alone."[13]

The irony of my views on this topic isn't lost on me, as someone who received a "Genius Grant" from the MacArthur Fellows Program. But my work is actually a powerful example of creativity beyond the individual. With Grandma Alice, I asked questions, she shook her finger or rolled her eyes, and together we told a story that neither of us could have told alone. I didn't create the story of Fred Astaire and Gina Autry that emerged in the locked Alzheimer's unit in a Milwaukee nursing home. I simply invited the story into being. As an artist primarily centered in theater, I can't make art without actors, directors, designers, and audiences. As a community-engaged artist, I am a facilitator of other people's creative expression. I have no studio—no lab in which to take brilliant solo creative leaps forward. My lab might be a nursing home and my collaborators all those who pass through the doors; or my lab might be a Meals on Wheels program and my fellow creators all those who deliver and receive the meals. Gene Cohen, whose ideas are certainly entangled with my own, writes that "our creativity shapes our relationships, and our relationships then become the context of our creativity."[14] I go even further. Creativity itself is born in relationships.

But telling the story of cocreation has always been a challenge. After my twelve weeks at the Marian Franciscan Center nursing home, I came away with a dozen vivid, poetic, haunting stories that I turned into a play. The characters from the stories came alive on stage, and in postshow discussions, we talked about how shifting from memory to imagination can open worlds of expression and connection. I remember sitting with a reporter trying to convey the backstory. The stories were created collaboratively with elders in a nursing home, I told the reporter. I simply facilitated them. The play itself was created collaboratively during the rehearsal process, shaped by the actors and director. I served as the writer, capturing and shaping the best bits out of rehearsal. I worked hard to emphasize the many hands at work on the play. But when the article came out, it had a big picture of me and told the story as though I had made it all happen myself. Thousands of years of stories about protagonists and heroes are hard to resist.

Perhaps this relational part of creativity is what is drawn out by putting it next to the word "care"? In this context, I have found everyone is able to embrace their creativity. But to tease out this puzzle, we must first understand the word "care" itself.

What Is Care?

If creativity is romanticized as an act of individual genius that yields a valuable product, care is largely understood as its opposite—an act of selflessness. In the case of caring for frail elders at the end of their lives, care can also be seen as futile and thankless. Definitions of care pepper writing across disciplines from philosophy to psychology, from social work to nursing and medical training. But I found no integrated definition. When the term appears in the field of aging, "care" tends to be described in the language of emergency and economics: as a financial and emotional burden that will bankrupt individuals and governments; emotionally burn out family and professional caregivers alike; and bleed productivity as workers take time to provide care for family members. In this light, care seems to be a black hole into which everything—money, work, meaning, our very beings— falls.

The various definitions of "care" that I found break along two fronts, physical and emotional,[15] and individual and reciprocal. Physical care often asks us to do things that make us queasy at best, nauseated or physically drained at worst. These are usually things to do with the body and its functions, around which have developed centuries of hiding and shaming practices. Smells. Sounds. Wiping. Emotional care is less dependent on proximity. Simple things like listening and attention can be a salve against loneliness and despair, ensuring that a person can flourish regardless of physical challenges. Of course, physical and emotional care are entwined. It can take significant emotional work to navigate the breaching of privacy and consent that physical care demands. When we are asked to take on new care responsibilities, the weight of memories of familial roles and expectations turned on their heads can add to the emotional labor of care. My otherwise hyperrational father became visibly upset, for example, when our conversation moved toward what Mom's dementia diagnosis might eventually demand from him in terms of physical care. "I won't wipe her, I'm sorry, I just won't," he said. Mom looked aghast. "I don't *want* you to wipe me!"

Part of Dad's agitation about wiping was surely locked into deeply ingrained gender roles. Most care professions are the terrain of women's labor, from nursing and social work to teaching and direct home care or nursing assistance, and are accompanied by the low wages and devaluing that seem to follow women's work into every field. Direct care workers are notoriously underpaid and commonly lack health care coverage for their own needs. Feminist scholars, activists, and organizers like Ai-jen Poo and the National Domestic Workers Alliance are pushing back against this devaluing of the labor of care in both wages and popular representations like movies and television. Arthur Kleinman, a psychiatrist with personal experience caring not just for patients but also for his wife, who experienced Alzheimer's disease, is pushing for a more comprehensive theory of care that elevates its value. Kleinman sees care "first and foremost as a developmental process that, whatever its biological basis, is learned and practiced as part of personal development, social cultivation, and maturation of our sensibilities and capabilities."[16] Care, in other words, can be imagined as the highest expression of human potential.

Like creativity, care has long been framed with the lens of the individual. "Care" referred to the actions of the caregiver, whether a spouse or a nurse, a home care worker or a surgeon. But focusing on the caregiver alone creates what I call the "empty-vessel" model of care. One person with a full vessel pours him- or herself into the other, empty vessel. This is the tragic-hero story of self-sacrifice: a recipe for caregiver burden and burnout. An empty vessel cannot refill itself. "Self-care" emerges in this model, with warnings to caregivers not to empty themselves fully but to take time to refill themselves. I understand the need to disrupt the empty-vessel model before caregivers deplete themselves and wind up sick. But this notion of "self-care" has always struck me as yet another layer of duty for the caregiver. Now caregivers must see to the needs of other people and also to themselves. If there were room in daily life to talk about caregiving, and if the work of care were valued, support structures to ensure that caregivers are cared for might well follow.

In the reciprocal model, on the other hand, care emerges in the relationship between partners. In this model, rather than emptying oneself into another person, both care partners are imagined to receive benefits. Care is an exchange. Research supports this view, but negative stories about caregiving are so prevalent that positive benefits can be hard to imagine. Studies on the positive aspects of care found that caregivers for people with Alzheimer's described feeling a sense of growth and purpose; growing closer to their care partner and family; learning how to laugh at difficulties; learning to let go of things they couldn't control.[17]

There are, of course, situations in which one care partner is resistant to care. Eva Feder Kittay, who writes about caregiving from the thick experience of caring for her daughter with profound disabilities and for elder relatives, takes a lesson from what she saw as her failure to care for a "cranky" uncle and a bitter mother. Even if Kittay's daughter couldn't verbalize her acceptance of care, her body responded. But her mother was different. "My mother's stubborn refusal and bitterness at the loss of capacities convinced me that care is not care until it is completed in the other." When someone does not take up our offering of care, care is not complete. "Without uptake, no matter our good intentions, our efforts are not care," writes Kittay.[18]

The fierce pressure to disguise evidence of aging and the stigma that shrouds dependency keep us isolated and ill prepared for stepping into caregiving roles. Too many caregivers are laboring alone and unsupported because they don't recognize themselves as caregivers, or because they hide away out of shame or the belief that they are protecting someone's dignity. This shame and silence can also breed depression and bitterness that Kittay describes as haunting her mother. How might we imagine being a good recipient of care? What might be the exchange of gifts between care partners? How to ensure both feel dignity? Support? Growth? While the model of reciprocal care has emerged in the last several years, there has been little conversation about what it might mean to be a good *recipient* of care and how we might learn or pass along such models. The day after my father burst forth with his discomfort about the possibility of having to provide physical care for my mom, we three were gathered in the tiny living room of their north-woods cabin. I was sitting behind them at the dining room table, out of view, when I observed my mother quietly reach out for my father's hands. He took them. "Have I told you how grateful I am for you?" she asked him softly. "Yes," he said, eyes welling, "You have." For a brief few years after college and before she started to have children, my mother was a social studies teacher. Now she is teaching both me and my father, even in her time of accumulating losses. She is giving us the incredible gift of modeling how to receive care.

"Creative care." What happens when these two words come together, dragging with them decades of preconceived ideas and assumptions? The tension between the words calls attention to the generative nature of one and the depleting qualities of the other. By its very definition, creativity is new and valued. Care seems the opposite, defined by loss, devalued at every turn, pulling down economic productivity and inhibiting generativity. Creativity is the place we want to be. Care is the place we're forced to go, sometimes kicking and screaming. Yet when we bring them together, the tension between them vibrates with possibility.

That tension can help us envision and shape a world in which care partners invite each other into meaning-making, together adding something new and valuable to the world—a world where growth is possible even in the deepest loss and all the way to the end of life. Bringing the words together helps us imagine and shape a world where care is reciprocal healing, where loss is no longer a black hole that consumes everything around it but instead can invite us to become our best selves—a world where creativity is assumed to emerge in relationship with caregiving and is the better for doing so. Bringing these two concepts together makes me question how each has functioned separately for so long—at least since the formalization of medicine and medical training in the nineteenth century.[19] Where has creativity been practiced? By whom? Where has care been practiced? By whom? Might places of creativity and culture-making also become places of healing? How might places of healing open themselves to culture- and meaning-making? Real meaning that resonates with and emerges from both care partners—not meaning that is prescribed by one for the benefit of the other.

When I was a kid, maybe ten years old, I would play outside for as long as I could. I remember there was a row of bushes down the hill along the side of our house. One of my favorite games was to burst through two of those bushes and into the open field next door. Each time I did it, I imagined a different location in the world, with a different sick animal that needed my help. Boom! I was on the savannah in Africa, tending to a sick giraffe. Boom! Alaska, rushing to aid a wounded otter. Boom! The north woods of Wisconsin, where a porcupine badly needed my attention. When I came inside from playing, my mom—I imagine her at the sink, fixing dinner—would simply ask me, "Which animals did you help today?" My mother, who loved gardening, hiking, painting, and writing.

What questions will I ask her? What questions will draw on who she is and invite her creativity?

The imagination can transport and transform us. Individually, in relationship to each other, and in our communities. Yet so much talk about creativity can intimidate. When I ask people whether they are creative, as I have done in workshops for years, nine times out of ten they back away with an apologetic "I can't draw." Or "I can't sing anymore." This might happen because being "creative" is seen as something someone says *about you*, like being handsome or clever, not something someone claims about themselves. But it is also possible that somewhere along the line, creativity has become a rare currency, a precious attribute associated with the few: the elite, the artist, the tech start-up CEO. It is my aim to bring creativity back home where it belongs. Back into the micromoments of our days when we can make meaning simply by noticing the angle of light as it pours through a window, the pattern of vowels on a billboard, the overlapping rhythms of Muzak and fingers tapping on a keyboard in a waiting room. It is my aim to remind us that human beings are innately creative and that inviting our fellow human beings to express themselves creatively, to cocreate, is itself an act of care, an expression of love.

After all my exploring and defining, I like the terms together. Creative care. It is more than medicine. It is more than the arts. It is more than therapy, but it has measurable therapeutic benefits. At its heart, creative care is not really about painting or singing, although those things certainly happen. Creative care is an agreement between people to imagine themselves, each other, and their worlds a little differently. It is an invitation to shape the world together. For people denied the tools for world-shaping, this invitation can be a profound and life-changing act of healing.

Exactly how does one go about inviting another person into an act of cocreation? After years of doing so and watching others do so, I see now that the invitation is deceptively simple. The steps are clear, even fun. But nearly each one runs counter to instinct in the hypercognitive, fast-paced, and tech-fawning contemporary moment. What are those elements? And how could they possibly be powerful enough to resist the temptation to turn over care to robots so we can get back to our computers and phones? In each chapter that follows, I focus on a core element of creative care; share stories of that element in action; and offer suggestions for how these elements might make their way into the daily lives of caregivers, family, and friends.

CHAPTER 4

"Yes, and . . ."

Imagine two performers on stage. One says "The toilet is broken! But all the plumber brought was . . ." The other performer embraces the world her partner has created and builds on it: "Half a pastrami sandwich and his standard poodle." Now it's the first player's turn to embrace the new information and see what a plumber might do with half a pastrami sandwich.

For those in theater, "Yes, and" is a phrase like "hello" or "good morning." When someone says it, you know what it means, and you know what to do. In the theater world, "Yes, and" has become a reflex. It is the core tenet in improvisation of all kinds. It means intensely observing and sensing what is happening around you, accepting it, and adding to it in a positive way.

"Yes, and" is not a natural, human response to the world around us. Observation, yes. Human beings are primed to be alert to our surroundings. But the first human response to new input is more often to say *no*. Saying no means we don't need to shift our position. Saying no eliminates risk of change. Saying yes, on the other hand, means we agree to accept something that might demand a considerable shift out of our comfort zone. In "Yes, and," we agree to shift our position with the knowledge that the other person will also say yes and add positively to our contribution. Saying "Yes, and" is an agreement between two people to play with and care for each other. It is, in essence, a performance of care.

Improvisation is as old as theater itself. Its roots trace back to ancient farces, on through to Italian street theater in the middle ages. "Yes, and" was codified in the work of theater artist Viola Spolin in the 1950s and became more widely known and used when she published *Improvisation for the Theater* in the 1960s. Spolin's son was a founding member of The Second City in Chicago, the famous home of countless lauded performers from Dan Aykroyd and John Belushi to Mike Myers and Tina Fey. The field became well established as groups like Comedysportz and the Upright Citizens Brigade created their own techniques and franchises across the United States. Improv techniques are finding their way into businesses, classrooms, and health-care settings as a way to increase flexibility, creativity, and presence in increasingly distracting environments.

Having played countless theater improvisation games in high school and college, "Yes, and" was in my toolbox when I began to engage with elders more regularly. "Yes, and" was the reason I could have a conversation with my grandmother who couldn't speak. She gave me the sound of "tsssss," a shake of her crooked finger, and a soulful opening and closing of her eyes. I accepted this communication and added questions that eventually led us to a shared story.

"Yes, and" was the reason the group of elders at the Marian Francis-can Center could tell a forty-five-minute story about Fred Astaire, the cowboy, that was filled with song, laughter, and occasional non-sense words. As a facilitator, "Yes, and" enabled me to accept what was offered and invite the group to add to it in positive ways.

In care settings, "Yes, and" can feel like a radical act, especially with people who have dementia. "Yes, and" can feel like the exact *wrong* thing to do. In the first story sessions I facilitated in a Milwau-kee adult day center, a staff member warned me that there would be resistance among staff to affirming the reality of a person with demen-tia: "We're trained *not* to do this," she said. When someone with de-mentia says something that we know is not true, the impulse is to gently correct them, as if a calm recitation of facts can heal a wounded brain. But we can't fix dementia by rebuilding the facts of someone's life brick by brick. All that does is create a brick wall between us. "Yes, and" helps us walk around the wall to find each other in a place where imagination, shared experience, and emotional truth can bond us.

Take Charlie Farrell, for example. I met Dr. Farrell when he at-tended a TimeSlips training workshop in 2005. His wife, Carolyn, was in the second year of her journey with dementia, and Charlie, a retired physician, was caring for her at home. He'd heard a story about TimeSlips on National Public Radio while he was driving, and when he got home he made a plane reservation to fly from Cleveland to Milwaukee to attend the training. Charlie has a serious and effi-cient demeanor. I remember admiring his posture—forever hearing my grandmother's voice echoing in my ear, scolding me for slouch-ing. I had structured the training workshop to slowly invite people into feeling confident in expressing their own creativity. It took me a while to realize just how deeply some people believe they are not creative. Opening up to play can feel remarkably uncomfortable to people who've been told and become convinced that creativity is not part of every human being's capacity. So through the course of two or three creative exercises, I wasn't surprised to see Charlie's shoulders relax a little. But then, as we shifted into the part of the training where we practice "Yes, and," meeting the person where they are and accepting what they are saying for its emotional truth, Charlie started to look pale. I remember that it was noticeable enough for me to stop in the middle of the training.

"Are you okay?" I asked.

"Yes," he said quietly. "I'm just realizing that I've been driving my wife crazy for the last two years."

For two years, every time Carolyn was confused about something, saying the wrong word, blanking on a name, or mistaking one person for another, Charlie would correct her: "No honey, she's not your sister, this is our daughter. She was born in . . . " This calm recitation of facts, this methodical building of the brick wall of fact, is familiar to anyone who has lived with dementia in their lives.

After the training, Charlie went home and fully embraced "Yes, and." "I realized it was really just a very effective way for two people to communicate," he told me. He and Carolyn used to go for walks in their neighborhood. They would stop at a house, and he would say, "Tony's house looks nice." But Carolyn would look lost. She didn't know who Tony was.

"So I just asked, 'What does this look like? What do you see?' She said she saw a dog in the flowerpot. And I realized that we could communicate about a lot of things that she had just a partial memory about," said Dr. Farrell.

Charlie and Carolyn's daughter Katie quickly picked up on the approach. When Carolyn would stare at the ketchup at the dinner table and say, "Pass the . . . " Katie would simply ask, "What do you want to call it?"

"Red sauce."

"Then red sauce it is."

"Yes, and" affirms the person's reality and gives the person the power to name, shape, and respond to his or her world with the tools that the person has. "Yes, and" teaches and rewards flexibility for both sides of the care partnership. But letting go of those factual bricks can be very difficult. Even though the "reality orientation" approach—quite literally reminding a person of the facts of the moment—is not as commonly taught today as it was in the 1980s, taking that approach remains a powerful impulse. For family members, it can be especially difficult to say yes to the current situation of the person with dementia. I certainly don't want to say "Yes!" to the fact that my mother has Alzheimer's. It can sting to say yes to misspoken words or the blanks where my name should be. I want her to be whole. I yearn to be the cared for. But the power of "Yes, and" to open up a world where we can connect emotionally will not work if we say "Yes, *but* . . ." or simply say no.

Take Tony, for example. I met Tony and his wife in the basement of a synagogue on the Upper East Side of New York City. This was one of the two adult day sites in New York where I was trying to replicate the story circles. With the support of the Brookdale National Group Respite program, Elizabeth Hartowicz welcomed a small group of elders with dementia two days a week for a couple of hours of activities and snacks. There were no windows, but the space had an air of grandness to it, as we gathered chairs in a circle at the bottom of an elegant staircase and atrium. The respite program was designed as a way to give caregivers a break, but they would often gather and sit with us, happy to see their loved one respond to the group.

Tony's wife told us that he had been a high-powered Madison Avenue guy. Elizabeth and I knew him as quiet and cautious, but with a spark that we hoped we could figure out how to release. To this one particular meeting I had brought a picture of a hand-drawn cowboy and horse taken from an old advertising campaign that I'd found on a postcard rack somewhere in lower Manhattan.

"What do you see?" I asked, the simplest of opening questions.

"That's a cowboy, isn't it, Tony?" said his wife, who sat next to him in the story circle. "Tony was in advertising for many years, right, Tony?"

I tried again, focusing my attention on the storytellers with dementia.

"What do you see? You can say anything you want, and we'll put it in the story."

The answers started to unfurl from the group.

"He is a handsome man," one of the ladies noted.

"The man and the handsome horse are making love," said another.

"A horse! My, my, my," added Tony's wife.

Tony was notably silent.

"No . . . they aren't making love, they are too much in the open," offered another storyteller.

"He is serenading the horse, singing a cowboy song," said another.

I asked the group what song they wanted him to be singing. They thought for quite a while.

Then Tony offered, "Get along, get along, get along . . ."

We were thrilled to hear his voice, to watch him risk naming a song, even if it was a fragment.

But then his wife corrected him. "You mean 'Git Along, Little Dogies.'" You could see the spark in his eyes go out.

The story evolved into an amazing tale of Thomas Rex the cowboy, a handsome man who is attracted to beautiful women ("like us," said one of the ladies) and his horse Godfrey, or God for short. God is a talking horse, they said. He's been trained.

But Tony never spoke again in the story. He'd been pulled out of "Yes," and into the world of corrections: "No, you mean . . ."

He is a handsome man.

The man and the handsome horse are making love.

A horse! My, my, my.

No . . . they aren't making love, they are too much in the open.

He is serenading the horse, singing a cowboy song.

(Singing) "Get along, get along, get along . . ."

They live in the west country.

They keep moving.

The cowboy is a married man, but he's very available.

He is attracted to beautiful women like us.

He is whatever age we want him to be.

He's probably around 28.

The horse thinks he's a good guitar player.

He's not riding the horse right now, but he does sometimes.

The horse's name is Godfrey, whoops, Godfreya.

The man's name is Thomas Rex.

They go by Tom and God.

*Tom and God are inseparable. They are buddies. They even sleep to-
gether, in the barn of course—it's much roomier.*

The cowboy is also singing "Daisy, Daisy, give me your answer do . . ."

God is a talking horse.

He's been trained.

If someone you love has dementia, the impulse to protect and re-
build memory can be almost irresistible. Caregivers describe grieving
dozens of little losses every day, of words, shared memories and roles
played in each other's lives, in the course of a slow progression toward
their loved one's eventual passing. Correcting the mistakes and filling in the pauses can feel like preserving the person's dignity and
valiantly refusing the progression of the disease. But correcting and
filling in is also refusing the person's expressions, which can shut the
person down entirely. Saying "No, you mean . . ." ends up being a
refusal of the person as he or she is now.

Saying "Yes, and" can enable both the caregiver and the person we
love to open to new experiences. Roger's wife had a very different
response from Tony's. Roger had been a postal carrier who loved ban-
tering and sharing stories with the people on his route. "He was always a storyteller," I remember his wife telling me. Even after he
retired, he was the heartbeat of the family, telling stories at gatherings and keeping everyone laughing. When Roger developed symptoms of dementia, the stories and jokes stopped. As it became
increasingly difficult to string the right words together, and as his
joke-telling rhythm faltered, Roger grew quiet. I was just starting the
story sessions at Luther Manor's adult day center in Milwaukee when
the local news came and filmed a session. Roger's wife saw the clip on
the evening news and called the next day. The next week, they drove

an hour to get to the program, and Roger became a star in the group. "You can say anything you want, and we'll add it to the story," was enough to encourage him to risk releasing a broken word into the room. When the student facilitators and I entered the room each week, Roger was beaming. He took special pride in making up inventive names for characters and engaging others in the process. There are many magical moments from storytelling with Roger, but perhaps my favorite was a story we were telling inspired by an image of a young, native Alaskan boy with sled dogs and a whip.

"What do you see?" we asked.

Unable to come up with the word, one of the storytellers made the sound of a whip.

Another said the word "whip."

"It looks like a snake, ready to bite him in the you know where," said Roger, eyes sparkling.

When we repeated the story, Roger said, "Did I say that?"

"Why, yes, you did Roger," said Nicole, a student facilitator.

"I was misproprusing," he said, grinning.

One storyteller thought the boy, whom Roger named Dimrock, looked hungry.

"He has his meals—serviced to him," said Roger, struggling to express the concept.

"By . . . by . . . by—"

Vera, two seats down the circle, leaned forward and said, "Meals on Wheels."

The group erupted in laughter.

Roger was elated. "Hey!" he said, "I knew that woman was alive over there! And that she'd say something really terrific!"

"Yes, and" enabled Roger to be a storyteller again, and to encourage others to do the same.

Like creativity, improvisation is having a moment. Established improvisation companies are applying the core tenets of improv to education, business, and health care. There are multiple improvisation training programs for caregivers. Karen Stobbe and Mondy Carter, who met (and married) at ComedySportz in Milwaukee, began applying improv to dementia care back in 1998 when Karen's father increasingly struggled with the symptoms. "It was natural for us because that's what we did for a living," said Stobbe. "My dad was an architect and a veteran, but he never ever talked about the war," said Stobbe. "Suddenly, with dementia, he wanted to talk about it." They went with it. Her father had been a bombardier, cramped in a tiny section of the plane, dropping bombs. Karen's brother brought in an old refrigerator box, and they encouraged their father to show them what it was like. "He drew every gauge and switch in that little compartment," said Karen. "It was incredible."

Karen worked with TimeSlips in the first adult day center trainings in Milwaukee, later joining the staff at Luther Manor and going on to build her own improvisation training program, In the Moment. "I still think there is no better way to teach communication," she said. Karen told me a story that illustrated her point. It happened when she was offering storytelling sessions at a Catholic nursing home as part of a research project testing the impact of the TimeSlips approach in twenty nursing homes. Each week Karen gathered together the elders, and each week a woman wheeled her husband into the room, said something to him, and kissed him on the forehead, and within minutes he would fall asleep. Karen was determined to understand what was happening, so she positioned herself by the couple one week. Leaning down, the wife said, "I don't know why they want you to do this, this is your nap time. And you can't tell stories." The next week Karen met the couple at the door and offered to wheel him in for her. Miraculously, he didn't fall asleep. "It took a few weeks," said Karen, "but eventually, he opened up." They were telling a story inspired by an old black-and-white image of a man jumping over a canyon, from one high rock to another. "What do you want to say happens?" asked Karen. The man held up two fingers above his head and brought them down slowly as if to demonstrate falling. "He made a squealing-screaming sound all the way down," said Karen, "until he hit the bottom, then he said 'Oh, shit.'" He seemed rather pleased with himself until he realized that he was surrounded by nuns. He flushed and apologized. One of the nuns leaned over and said, "Oh don't be silly. I've heard much worse." The group laughed and, according to Karen, "then he really started to open up and play."

Improvisation classes for families with dementia are slowly finding their way into more communities, like ImprovBoston, or Chicago's Memory Ensemble, a collaboration between the Lookingglass Theatre and the Mesulam Center for Cognitive Neurology and Alzheimer's Disease at Northwestern University's Feinberg School of Medicine. Caring Across Generations, The Second City, and the Cleveland Clinic have teamed up to teach and assess improv techniques for caregivers, as have the University of Iowa and Dr. Jade Angelica's Healing Moments. The programs vary in duration (two-day intensives or six- or eight-week sessions) but follow the same basic elements, focusing on improving observation skills; learning to use verbal and non-verbal communication; exercising patience (often through mindfulness);

being present in the moment; and, of course, saying "Yes, and"—accepting what is given to you and engaging positively. Research has been tricky. Listening to the laughter and seeing the faces of participants tells one story. The data from surveys for things like depression, anxiety, and burden have yet to budge the stubborn needle on these complex, chronic conditions, for both sides of the care partnership.

But you cannot deny the joy. You cannot deny the endless examples of both caregivers and elders finding and connecting with each other. "Yes, and" becomes a window. The facilitator's role is to open that window—in some cases pry it open—and hold it open, sometimes for weeks, until the person with dementia can step through it into expression, connection, meaning, and joy.

In a bustling and beloved Milwaukee pizza restaurant, more than a dozen people from three strands of my family joined for one last night of Thanksgiving weekend festivities. I sat next to Mom in the center of the long table. My sister sat across from us. Toward the end of the meal, Mom turned to me, gently put her hand on my shoulder, and asked, "Where's Annie?"

She was concerned. Maybe they had forgotten to invite me.

I felt the rush that millions of people who love someone with dementia must feel.

There it is, I thought. The lacuna where I should be.

I saw the concern on her face. I imagined seeing the neuron in her brain—the one responsible for getting the information to the right place—sputter and collapse.

"Do you mean Ellen? She went to the bathroom," I offered. Explaining why there was a blank chair where my sister was just minutes ago.

Mom held my eyes for a moment. The restaurant spun with laughter and silver pizza trays.

A smile slowly broke across her face.

"You're right there," she said, almost marveling at the rescue of information that some other neuron had performed.

"Yes," I said. "I'm right here. And I love you."

NOTES FOR CAREGIVERS:

✦

"Yes, and" at Home

If you are caring for someone with dementia at home, perhaps the most important step of "Yes, and" is to notice when you are about to say no. In what kinds of situations do you say no? And how might "Yes, and" open them up?

Is the person misremembering something or someone?

Try saying yes to the emotions of the moment and ask the person how he or she feels about it.

"I need to go to the doctor" **(when she was at the doctor last week).**

"Is something bothering you?"

"How do you feel about the doctor?"

"Where is my mother?" **(when his mother has long since passed away).**

"Are you thinking of her? Can you tell me a story about her?"

"Let's write her a letter" (or "Let's draw a picture").

Is the person doing something wrong, like putting dish soap in the washing machine?

"That's dish soap. Should we make bubbles with it?"

"That's dish soap. How many dishes do you think we've washed in our lives?"

Is the person making a repetitive movement, like folding or rolling paper?

"Let's see how many of those we can do together!"

"What can that rolled paper be? A telescope?

If the person is doing something dangerous like opening the car door while the car is moving, saying no might be your very best option in the moment. But saying "Yes, and" can follow on its heels:

"Let's make the sound of the car."

"Let's sing together."

"We aren't there yet. Let's say the name of the place we are going in ten different ways."

CHAPTER 5

Beautiful Questions

I want to beg you, as much as I can, dear sir, to be patient toward all that is unsolved in your heart and to try to *love the questions themselves* like locked rooms and like books that are written in a very foreign tongue. Do not now seek the answers, which cannot be given you because you would not be able to live them. And the point is, to live everything. *Live* the questions now. Perhaps you will then gradually, without noticing it, live along some distant day into the answer.

RAINER MARIA RILKE,
Letters to a Young Poet

Back in the chaotic dining room of the Marian Franciscan Center, I got lucky. Driven by desperation after six weeks of failure to draw out the expressions of the residents who generously put up with my creative fumbling, I held up a picture of the Marlboro Man and asked, "What do you want to name him?"

That question unlocked forty-five minutes of laughter and singing, of joy and surprise. What was it about that phrasing that was so different from what I'd been doing for six weeks?

Questions are remarkably flexible things. A question can strangle response—forcing it into a tight yes-or-no option or coating it with intimidation so respondents twist their words into what they hope is the "right" answer. On the other hand, a question can invite a person into contemplation without worry over right or wrong—an act of expression that is wholly the person's own. This latter form is what I have come to call a "beautiful question," one that invites the asker and the listener onto a shared path of discovery. There is no right or wrong answer to a beautiful question. There is only exploration and expression. In my work with TimeSlips to train people in improvisational storytelling, we used to call these "open-ended questions," because they don't have a specific answer. But I have come to see the crafting and asking of such questions as an art, carefully shaping the question to inspire the listener to embark on a journey toward an answer that is ongoing—that is, in fact, the process of articulating who we are.

My interpretation and understanding of the beautiful question were inspired in part by an interview I heard between Krista Tippett (of the podcast *On Being*) and the poet David Whyte, who relayed a story of his friend and poet John O'Donohue:

And John used to talk about how you shaped a more beautiful mind, and that it's an actual discipline, no matter what circumstances you're in. The way I interpreted it was the discipline of asking beautiful questions, and that a beautiful question shapes a beautiful mind. And so the ability to ask beautiful questions, often in very unbeautiful moments, is one of the great disciplines of a human life. And a beautiful question starts to shape your identity as much by asking it as it does by having it answered.

Tippett responds, "So you call forth something beautiful by asking a beautiful question?" "Yes," says Whyte. "Yes, you do."[1]

O'Donohue, Tippett, and Whyte are referring to the questions one asks of oneself. But you can call forth something beautiful from another person as well. To ask a beautiful question as an invitation to another is to believe that the listener can do this and that the asker will receive and honor the listener's answer. So the beautiful question is an invitation both to selfhood and to community simultaneously. This is an incredibly powerful tool for those who become stigmatized through frailty, aging, loneliness, or dementia. This tool is also incredibly powerful for those who love people who have been edited or who edit themselves into silence and who yearn to connect with those silent loved ones but don't know how.

That disconnection can be devastating. Walter has taken care of his wife, Arlie, all through her experience of dementia. A successful businessman in a tight community of friends and family in northern Wisconsin, Walter adjusted to many caregiving duties but was blindsided by the isolation. "I'll tell you," he wrote, "nothing is more painful than when your friends just stop calling." Stan Berg, who cared for his wife with Alzheimer's for more than a decade, described the phenomenon as "The Law of Disappearing Friends." In a blog post about his experiences, he included a chart showing a steady decline in friendships as the disease progressed. New friendships can be formed with people in support groups who, as Berg described it, "have their eyes wide open" to the disease. But old friends, who keep so much of our shared memory, too commonly fall away over time.[2]

There are myriad reasons that people fall away from friends or family with dementia: fear, grief, and a genuine uncertainty of what to say or how their presence might be helpful. But once loneliness sets in, the feeling itself can be stigmatizing, making it even more difficult to form those crucial social networks and emotional relationships upon which our well-being depends.[3] Caregivers in the grip of grief might also hold tightly in their minds to the person as he or she once was. Grief and a gut instinct to reorient a person with dementia to "reality" push against our ability to broadly embrace "Yes and" (or improvisation) in care relationships. To invite people to shape and offer beautiful questions similarly asks caregivers to swim against the current. Caregivers are commonly trained to offer yes-or-no questions or limited options to people with memory loss to enable them to have a sense of choice without being overwhelmed. Do you want a cookie or pudding? Do you want to sit here or there? This tight phrasing is indeed efficient and can be used to guide everyday actions. But it won't open up a shared experience of meaning-making. For that, you need a beautiful question.

How exactly do these questions work? You can create questions about a prompt of any kind, like a bowl of fruit on the breakfast table, a view out the window, or an image from a magazine or greeting card. If we can imagine that original image of the Marlboro Man, these are questions I might use to open a world full of senses, emotions, people, and plot:

What do you see?

Where do you want to say this takes place?

When do you want to say it takes place?

What do you want to name him?

Who else might be there?

What do they like to do?

What do they do for a living?

What do they dream of?

How are they feeling?

What happened just before this moment?

What happens next?

One can spot a beautiful question because it gives the creative power to the listener, not the asker. If you pass by a window together, spot a scraggly pine tree, and ask, "Do you think that is Charlie Brown's Christmas tree?" your question is a demonstration of your creativity, not the listener's. Instead you might ask, "What do you see?" or "What do you imagine the sounds are outside?" or "If you could paint the tree, what colors would you use?" or "If you could name that tree, what would you want to name it?"

Beautiful questions can be shaped around a prompt, like the view out a window, or stand alone as a prompt themselves. Working with Sojourn Theatre on a project called Islands of Milwaukee in 2014, I learned the simple power of such questions, and now the TimeSlips website features a whole section called beautiful questions:

What do you treasure in your home and why?

What is your safe harbor?

What is courage?

Imagine seeing such a question, printed in bold letters on substantial paper. It's just a simple four-inch-by-six-inch card, but the poetic phrasing and vibrant design somehow catches on the routine of your day and unravels it just enough to make an opening, to invite you to think a little differently. Imagine such questions delivered with the Meals on Wheels program. Or by a volunteer who comes to sit with you for a bit in the afternoons.

For the Islands of Milwaukee project, which I describe more in chapter 11, Sojourn's Maureen Towey and I coordinated a team of artists to bring meaningful engagement to elders living alone. After shadowing Meals on Wheels drivers and studying the daily routines of volunteers and home care workers, we designed "questions of the day" to inspire people to see themselves and their surroundings with fresh eyes. Elders were invited to respond by phone or by writing on the card itself.

Ernest received his questions of the day through a daily phone call. A trained volunteer would check in with him once a day just to make sure Ernest, who lives alone, was okay. One day, after we'd been sending out questions for a couple of months, we got a phone message from Ernest. He said that when his volunteer first asked him these questions, he thought they were stupid. They both did. "But then," Ernest said, "she asked me 'What is your safe harbor?' and I thought—that's not a stupid question. That's an interesting question." He said his answer was his church. And he and his volunteer marveled that that was her answer as well. "So now," said Ernest on the voice mail, "I'd like to answer all your previous questions."

His message was more than thirty minutes long.

As part of the Islands of Milwaukee project, two of my students at the University of Wisconsin–Milwaukee (UWM), Sammy and Cu, arranged to visit June, a woman in her eighties who lived with her daughter. Because of her daughter's work schedule, June was alone most days and asked to receive companionship visits from a local nonprofit. Sammy was a musical theater major, who had come to the class in the hopes of learning how to engage her father, who had Alzheimer's. Cu was a theater major, looking for ways to use his craft for social good. Visiting once a week, they tried out several questions. It was when they asked, "What do you treasure in your home and why?" that sparks began to fly.

"Well, that would be my oven," said June.

An oven? Really? Not family photos, the Bible, or even "my dog"? These were the answers we heard over and over on the project voice mail or read in determined handwriting on the cards the Meals on Wheels drivers returned to us. But an oven? The two college students—who didn't cook—were puzzled. How could an oven be a treasure? They came to discover that June was a baker. Not professionally, but June loved to bake for family and had become known for it across the generations of children and grandchildren.

"When was the last time you baked?" wondered Sammy. June wasn't sure.

One beautiful question sparked an entire series.

"If you could bake anything right now, what would you bake?" asked Cu.

"My favorite. Almond cookies with banana frosting," said June.

"Does your oven work?" the students asked. June wasn't sure.

And finally, the best question of all: "Should we try it?"

It was a yes-or-no question, but it launched them even farther down the path of creativity.

Over the next couple of weeks, Sammy, Cu, and June found the recipe; gathered ingredients and baking pans; and baked almond cookies with banana frosting, which turns out to be regular frosting with banana flavoring. To deepen the meaningfulness of their project, they put three or four cookies in a baggie with a colorful, printed note. On one side was the recipe. On the other, a note that read, "These cookies are from June's oven, which she treasures. What do you treasure?" They gave the cookies to the Meals on Wheels drivers as a thank-you for their work.

Over the years at TimeSlips, we've honed and shaped many beautiful questions. There are questions that open what might otherwise be unremarkable passing moments: a stroll by the window, a silent ride in a slow elevator, a meal eaten in silence. A simple question can enchant such moments with imagination. There are questions that invite listeners to respond to images or other prompts (songs, objects, and so on). "What do you want to name him?" "Where do you want to say this is?" "What happened just before this moment? Just after?"

Then there are the thoughtful poetic questions that take us down a rabbit hole of wonderment. One of my favorites comes from a nursing home in Texas. Jamie Ward is a certified TimeSlips facilitator with Unity Theatre, which offers fourteen weeks of TimeSlips sessions as part of its senior adult outreach program. Jamie was starting sessions with a new group at the Brenham Nursing and Rehabilitation Center in Brenham, Texas. Rather than use one of the many image prompts on the TimeSlips website, Jamie thought she would try one of the beautiful questions: "If your feet could talk, what would they say?"

At the nursing home, just as Jamie was preparing to start her session, a woman rolled into the room with a big black brace on her left foot. "She appeared to be uncomfortable, solemn, and extremely quiet," Ward wrote me in an email describing the day. She almost changed the question because of the woman's situation but decided to push on. She was glad she did. The woman began to open to the process as she realized her thoughts were safe and accepted by the group. Asked, "What would your feet say?" the woman answered, "My nerves hurt deep down." Asked, "Where would your feet take you?" She said "Home. Home to my husband." The minute she voiced this, she started to tear up. Ward knelt by her and held her hand, and the entire group paused to honor her. "Then they went right on adding their own thoughts," Ward wrote. The next woman responded, "To Temple, Texas, to the cemetery where my parents and husband are buried . . . and I'd stay a little while." The group paused again to honor her response and hold the weight of the emotion. Then another woman broke the spell, chiming in with a joyful, "These feet can take me anywhere!" "It was really quite beautiful," wrote Ward.

If your feet could talk, they would say . . . ?

> I'm tired.
>
> I hurt.
>
> I want to skip.
>
> Take my shoes off!
>
> My nerves hurt deep down.
>
> Hot dogs!
>
> If my feet could thank me, they would say . . .
>
> Good shoes.
>
> Tennis shoes.

Air condition.

Thank you.

Put me in some warm water!

Relax.

Splash.

Going swimming!

Paddle.

Kick.

That's what helps us swim—paddling, moving our arms.

(*Singing*) These shoes are made for walking, and that's just what they'll do. One of these days these shoes are gonna walk all over you.

I think that just about does it (*laughing*).

Walking.

Too tight shoes.

Ow! Shoes don't fit.

Help!

My feet would take me . . .

In the water.

To work. Both of my feet.

Home, to my husband (*tearing up*).

Home.

Anywhere!

To Temple, Texas, to the cemetery where my parents and husband are buried . . . and I'd stay a little while (*dreamily*).

These feet can take me anywhere!

I would go see the world! I would travel and travel and travel . . . and see Europe! And I would show my family all of the world that God has shown to me.

To church. Every Sunday.

Church.

Beautiful feet.

Baby feet.

Nice.

Clean, smooth.

I wouldn't say mine are pretty feet! (*laughing*)

Authors: Doris, Genevieve, Pat, Delores, Phyllis, Allyne, Patsy, and Darlene

For people experiencing dementia, answering a question *wrong* can have dire consequences. If their answer reveals that their condition has worsened, it might mean they have to move. It might mean they have to take pills that have serious side effects. It might mean a change in diagnosis that scares off the few people who keep visiting. I have seen this in my mother, who bristled at having to take a three-hour neurodiagnostic test. Piles and piles of questions exhausted her and threatened her with stigma, with the possibility of having to move and sell a beloved house, and with forever changing her relationship with my dad. Diagnostic questions, designed to seek out and identify the losses revealed by brain changes, are not beautiful. They feel like sharp-toothed traps.

But what if those tests contained a few beautiful questions? Questions that open a shared path to discovery and that reveal and exercise remaining strengths?

That is a beautiful question in and of itself.

NOTES FOR CAREGIVERS:

✦

Beautiful Questions
at Home

The first step is to learn what a closed question feels like, and when it is useful.

Closed questions have one or two answers at the most: This one or that one? Yes or no?

They are very useful when trying to encourage someone to make a task-based choice, like getting dressed or eating.

Beautiful questions are powerful in quiet moments of being, when we have the time and space to explore the world a bit.

A quiet moment looking out the window together can be transformed by beautiful questions.

What do you see?

What do you hear?

What do you feel?

What do you think that tree is thinking?

If the tree could talk, what might it say?

Quiet moments at the kitchen table are also ideal for opening the world with beautiful questions.

If we could invite someone to our table right now, whom would you invite?

What would you say to them?

What story do you have about them?

What would you feed them?

Beautiful questions can also help unlock an emotion or illuminate something that is bothering a person. If someone seems in pain, you can ask a beautiful question to understand more.

If your foot could talk, what would it say?

If your foot were a color, what color would it be? Why?

Beautiful questions can also engage the whole family.

Visit the Creativity Center on the TimeSlips website, timeslips.org, and see our list of questions. You can download and print them to use at home.

You can write or audio-record your answers online and share them with family and friends. You can invite faraway family to answer with you, too.

CHAPTER 6

Proof of Listening

No more fiendish punishment could be devised, were such a thing physically possible, than that one should be turned loose in society and remain absolutely unnoticed by all the members thereof. If not turned round when we entered, answered when we spoke, or minded what we did, but if every person we met "cut us dead" and acted as if we were non-existent things, a kind of rage and impotent despair would ere long well up in us, from which the cruelest bodily tortures would be a relief; for these would make us feel that, however bad might be our plight, we had not sunk to such a depth to be unworthy of attention at all.

WILLIAM JAMES,
The Principles of Psychology

Human beings are social creatures. We are social not just in the trivial sense that we like company, and not just in the obvious sense that we each depend on others. We are social in a more elemental way: simply to exist as a normal human being requires interaction with other people.

ATUL GAWANDE,
"Hellhole"

It's a little sign. You might miss it if you aren't looking for it. It's just a little clearing of the throat, a staccato series of tiny coughs. I heard it in nursing homes and assisted-living homes among people gathered for an activity. I heard it when I shadowed Meals on Wheels drivers, as people opened the doors to greet them. "(*Cough-cough-cough*) Hello!" I heard myself make the sound when I was writing my dissertation in a cabin in the woods and made my daily trek to the post office to see another human being. The sound is a sign that this is the first time a person has spoken that day. Maybe you've heard it. Maybe you've made the sound yourself.

In the many nursing homes I have visited, it is common to see people in their rooms, either alone or with a curtain pulled between the two beds. Or you might see a group of elders in wheelchairs gathered around the nurse's station, heads down, seemingly with no awareness of the people around them. Even during scheduled activity time, as elders sit in groups in a common area, there is often little interaction. I once visited a large nursing home with a group of student researchers to test a research protocol for observing engagement between staff and residents. Our plan was to code the type of interactions (social or physical; negative, neutral, or positive) during a ten-minute window of time—ten minutes on, ten minutes off—over a two-hour period. The students were nervous about being able to track all the interactions, especially during mealtimes and activity time. The students would begin coding when they observed a staff member interacting with a resident. Pencils up, ready, the students waited for the staff–resident interactions. The students saw staff passing by. They saw meals being handed out. They saw someone reading *Chicken Soup for the Soul* aloud to a room full of elders, most of whom were sleeping in their chairs.

The students saw staff come up from behind, say something aloud to a person without waiting for acknowledgment, grab the handles of the wheelchair, and wheel the person away. But the students could not actually say that they saw a staff member *engage* with a resident during an entire two-hour period. The students never started coding interactions. We had to revise the protocol.

I remember being profoundly moved when I read Atul Gawande's essay on solitary confinement in the *New Yorker* back in 2009. In it he traces the impact of intense isolation through early studies on baby monkeys and interviews with and research studies of long-term hostages, prisoners of war, and super-maximum-security (supermax) inmates.[1] The essay was fascinating and elegantly written, and when I started to read the symptoms of this extreme isolation, a light came on. Citing the work of Craig Haney, a psychology professor at the University of California, Santa Cruz, Gawande builds his case for the cruelty of isolation:

First, after months or years of complete isolation, many prisoners "begin to lose the ability to initiate behavior of any kind— to organize their own lives around activity and purpose," [Haney] writes. "Chronic apathy, lethargy, depression, and despair often result . . . . In extreme cases, prisoners may literally stop behaving," becoming essentially catatonic.

Second, almost ninety percent of these prisoners had difficulties with "irrational anger," compared with just three percent of prisoners in the general population. Haney attributed this to the extreme restriction, the totality of control, and the extended absence of any opportunity for happiness or joy.

In one study Gawande cites, electroencephalograms (EEGs) of prisoners kept in isolation revealed brain abnormalities similar to traumatic injury, after only a few months of isolation: Apathy. Lethargy. Depression. Anger attributed to extreme restriction and the extended absence of opportunity for happiness or joy. These words could describe nearly every nursing home I'd ever stepped foot in. Yet these words were attributed to dementia. Certainly, people with loving caregivers at home could experience these symptoms as well. But were some layers of these symptoms iatrogenic? Could we really tell the difference between symptoms caused by a changing brain and those caused by the environment of care? Could we legitimately say that some of our nursing homes and assisted-living or memory-care settings are actually keeping elders in group solitary confinement?

The call floating down the hallway of the nursing home where my grandmother lived—"Help me"—echoes still.

The need for meaningful engagement is clear. The previous two chapters, "Yes, and . . ." and "Beautiful Questions," provide a framework for and the entry point to that engagement. But none of it works if we don't listen. And we need not just to appear to listen but to offer *proof of listening* so that the person actually *feels heard*. Feeling heard can begin to crack the shell of isolation. Feeling heard consistently, over a period of time, can, according to Jill Stauffer, begin the long road to healing not just isolation or loneliness, but ethical loneliness— the feeling that one has been abandoned by humanity and civic society.[2]

How does one show proof of listening? Doing so begins with focus and observation. When I step into a group of elders, I am fully focused on them, and on reading communication in body language, facial expressions, what is said, and what is unsaid. Where are they sitting? How are they sitting? Is there tension in their faces? Their bodies? Second, I make sure that they can see and hear me as an equal. This means I kneel, crouch, or sit next to them if they are seated, and that I am making direct eye contact. If someone has difficulty hearing me, I ask if I can approach, and then speak directly into the person's ear. Third, I echo back what the person says to me—capturing both the verbal and the nonverbal, from gestures and sounds to facial expression and intent. Is the response meant to be funny? Sarcastic? Annoyed? Annoying? I also write down what people are saying so they can follow along and make changes if they wish. Fourth, I embrace silence. I will hold that silence for a long time, stopping just before it feels like I might be annoying the person, as in "Enough already, I'm not going to say anything." Focus. Be seen and heard. Echo back all responses. Embrace silence.

A few examples can help bring these steps alive. One particular story session comes to mind. It took place at Luther Manor's Adult Day Program in the quiet "skylight" room for people with memory loss. A handful of student facilitators joined me as I made my way around the semicircle of about ten people to welcome them to storytelling. Rose was a warm soul, always checking on people. She would wait patiently for us to start a story session at the day center. After the students settled in and asked their first questions, Rose jumped in. When one of the students asked, "What do you want them to eat?" Rose said, "Sweet and sour squirrel," enthusiastically. Kris followed up, trying her best to hide her incredulity.

"Sweet and sour squirrel casserole?"

"Yes," said Rose.

"Well, how might you make that?"

Rose proceeded to give step-by-step details for what was clearly a favorite recipe.

Kris repeated it all back to Rose, from the oversized sketch pad where Kris had written it all down. Rose followed along as Kris read.

"It's a sweet and sour squirrel casserole, with pine nuts and raisins."

"Right!"

"First you fry the squirrel, then you bake it," said Kris, making the same hand gestures that Rose had made, indicating a frying pan and then an oven dish. "In a light tomato sauce."

"Not too heavy," said both of them simultaneously—and Rose gave a warm, full-body laugh. Clearly Kris was listening.

Kris continued, "And it is served with a light orange wine."

"Right!" Rose said enthusiastically. "We make that. It's delicious."

And with each retelling of the story, Rose followed the recipe closely. Each time Kris repeated the recipe, Rose would check to make sure all the details were there. "Yes, a light tomato sauce," she confirmed. "Yummy, yummy. I'm getting hungry," she said with a grin.

As we finished the session and thanked the storytellers for all they had done and the gift of their time, energy, and creativity, Rose said:

"If you need a recipe, just call me."

Proof of listening gave Rose a sense of purpose. In an adult day program a thousand miles away, proof of listening drew Dorothy out of an anxious, repetitive loop. In the basement of the synagogue on the Upper East Side of Manhattan, a small group gathered in a circle of chairs at the bottom of the atrium. Dorothy wore a worried face.

The taut lines across her forehead and vague fear behind her eyes seemed to say, "How can this be?" "How did I get here?" But the only sounds that came from her mouth were "Ba ba ba ba." She only offered the sounds if someone asked her a question. "How are you today Dorothy?" might receive a "Ba ba ba ba ba" in return. Was there a pattern? Was it the same number of syllables each time? Was there a code we could crack? There didn't seem to be.

But the storytelling sessions were different. We welcomed the storytellers to the moment and assured them that they didn't need to remember anything. Elizabeth, who hosted the day center, and I offered a constant reminder that the storytellers could say anything they wanted and we would weave it into the story. We were just making up a story together after all. Dorothy had the same answer to every question, but Elizabeth and I echoed every response, the number of "Ba's," and the worry, wonder, or humor behind them. Did the inflection go up or down? I would look Dorothy in the eyes and repeat back what she had offered. "Ba ba ba ba ba ba?" I asked her. Yes, she nodded, and a light sparked somewhere deep behind her eyes. This became routine for a few weeks. But then something shifted. I asked the group what they wanted to name a character in the story.

"Ba ba ba ba ba Dorothy ba ba ba ba."

The entire group took a collective breath. I repeated what she had said back to her—trying to echo her as best I could but unable to separate a layer of giddiness from my own voice.

"Ba ba ba ba ba Dorothy ba ba ba ba?"

She beamed. Yes indeed. That would be the name of the character. Slowly and deliberately, she added, "Ba ba ba I love you ba ba ba."

I held her hands and echoed it back to her. Slowly, deliberately.

It wasn't a cure. It didn't fix any biomarkers of whatever was wreaking havoc in her brain. But Dorothy was heard. And she gave me the simplest, biggest gift in return. I cried the whole long subway ride home to Brooklyn.

Not all examples of the power of being heard are as profound as Dorothy's. I once facilitated a session in a care center in St. Paul, Minnesota, where about six elders in wheelchairs gathered around the flip chart I had set up in a corner of the room. I asked the usual, open-ended, beautiful questions. What do you want to name them? Where do you want to say they are? One gentleman spoke softly; I couldn't quite figure out what he was saying. I moved closer and asked him to repeat what he had said. They weren't words I recognized. I tried repeating them. He smiled broadly, correcting my pronunciation slightly. I tried again. He smiled his approval with a glint in his eyes. I wrote it down phonetically, unclear if it was an answer out of aphasia, a made-up word, or perhaps another language. People with dementia tend to retreat to the language they first learned. Was it Swedish? The care home had a strong Scandinavian heritage. The more I repeated the story, with his multiple contributions, the more I saw his smile grow, and spread across the circle of storytellers.

Then it dawned on me.

"I'm saying dirty words in Swedish, aren't I?"

He nodded, eyes sparkling.

"Does it bother any of you?" I asked the group. Clearly, no one was upset.

"Doesn't bother me," I shrugged. "I don't speak Swedish."

When Roger first started at the Luther Manor day center, he tested the process. Would we *really* echo back everything he said?

The prompt image was silly. It featured what I now know is a Shrove Tuesday tradition—a half dozen women were walking together outside, flipping pancakes in skillets. One of the student facilitators asked, "What do you want to say they are doing?" After a few responses of "flipping pancakes," Roger added, "Someone is throwing bits of dirty toilet paper at them."

I repeated it. "Someone is throwing bits of dirty toilet paper at them?"

"Yes," said Roger matter-of-factly. I had indeed gotten that right.

The group was not happy with the turn in the story.

"Ewww," said one woman. I echoed it back to her.

But I also reminded them that all answers are right. We're just making up a story together.

Each time we retold the story, I repeated Roger's line.

"'Someone is throwing bits of dirty toilet paper at them,' said Roger." And "Ewwww, Vera thought that was disgusting."

On one of the final retellings of the story, Roger stopped me after I had repeated his line.

"I don't want to say that anymore," he said.

"It's okay—you can say anything," I said.

"No, let's take that out."

And so I did, along with Vera's response.

Truly being heard made Roger hear and feel the impact of his words.

Truly being heard opened Dorothy to experiment with expression.

Truly being heard gave power to the Swedish gentleman, who I am guessing did not have much power in his daily life at the nursing home.

When I talk about this approach, people always ask whether there are situations in which people say things that I can't repeat. Over the past twenty years and during thousands of engagements, only twice could I not fully echo back what someone offered. In one instance, one woman used the worst word she could imagine, a sharp slap to the African-American caregivers interspersed throughout our group. It could be that she felt profoundly helpless and used the word to claw back some sense of power. It could be that she had always felt this way and felt no qualms about using the word now. It could be that the mysteries of the frontal lobe that controls social mores were betraying her—much as when prim and proper people begin to swear a blue streak as they journey through dementia. Whatever they were, the reasons were unknowable.

"I'm so sorry," I said. "I know I said that I would repeat anything you say, but that word hurts my heart and I just can't say it. Can you think of another word?"

She studied me carefully. I held her gaze and repeated my apology and request. She didn't offer another word in that moment. But she watched and listened carefully as we built the story together as a group.

The second instance was back on the upper east side of Manhattan, back in the basement of the synagogue. One woman who gathered with us each Tuesday was a mystery to me. Her white hair swirled upward, an elegant sweep tucked in with pins. She wore bright red lipstick and oversized black sunglasses. Someone prepared her for going out with incredible panache. She rarely spoke. When she did, it was almost always a flat refrain of "I want to die." The first time I heard it, my heart nearly broke. It was without energy, without emotion. Just a simple fact, as though she was saying her name. I looked to the other volunteers, but they were unfazed. I couldn't bring myself to repeat it. I simply held her hands. "Do you want to add that to the story?" I asked. A thin flat exhale carried the words out of her mouth. "I want to die." No, she didn't want to add it to our story, the story the group was building together. This *was* her story.

I want so badly to tell you that, like Dorothy, she added other words. But I don't think she ever did. She listened and watched from behind those dramatic black sunglasses. Perhaps her spirits lightened while the group laughed and sang. Perhaps not. But I wonder what would have happened if I had been brave enough to echo her response—to meet her emotions where they were, to see if I was getting it right. To give her the opportunity to confirm or reshape her response. To be heard.

Rachel Naomi Remen talks about "generous listening," when people respect what they receive with focus and attention.[3] Teachers talk about "authentic listening," learning to listen without judgment or preforming your response in your head as a person speaks. David Isay, founder of StoryCorps, says, "Listening is an act of love." I have come to call this act simply offering proof of listening. Whatever you want to call it, people should know that they've been heard. That their presence has registered. That they are not invisible. That their words and their being matter.

✦

Proof of Listening at Home

If you are caring for someone with dementia at home, proof of listening might be the simplest element of creative care to try.

People living with dementia commonly have trouble articulating their thoughts. Words seem to evaporate or jumble. The most common response is to ignore or rephrase for the person. But this response only further humbles and silences the person with dementia.

If someone says something that you don't understand or that doesn't make sense to you—for whatever reason—try echoing their response instead of correcting it.

Echo their words back to them. Echo their intention. Their pitch. Their facial expression. Ask them if you are getting it right. Is that what they said? Is that what they meant?

You can also echo gestures or movements for people who do not communicate verbally. Think of this as dancing, but you're letting the person with communication challenges lead.

While people still have expressive capacity, they might well rephrase or complete their thoughts or movements. Encouraged by the power of listening, they might try harder to communicate.

CHAPTER 7

Connecting to the Larger World

The self-transcendence of human existence. It denotes the fact that being human always points, and is directed, to something, or someone, other than oneself—be it meaning to fulfill or another human being to encounter. The more one forgets himself—by giving himself to a cause to serve or another person to love—the more human he is and the more he actualizes himself.

VIKTOR FRANKL,
Man's Search for Meaning

At the end of ten weeks of storytelling sessions at Luther Manor's day center, the student facilitators, center staff, and I put our heads together. What kind of celebration could we hold to honor the beauty of these stories and the effort of the storytellers? We decided on a party, of course. It would be at the end of the day so families could join us and then take loved ones home with them. We ordered food, made invitations, and gathered two dozen stories together into books. One of the students designed the cover—a colorful butterfly that appeared to take flight when the book was fully opened. Dick Blau, the photographer who had been shadowing the sessions for weeks, took portraits of all the storytellers, printed the portraits, and tucked a copy into the back of each of the storybooks. No one takes their pictures anymore, he told me. He wanted them to have a beautiful portrait of their "now."

On the day of the celebration, the center was packed with people. When everyone settled in, Beth Meyer Arnold, the director of the day center, and I gave some opening remarks, read a few of our favorite stories, and handed out the books to the families of the storytellers. When Beth handed the book to Roger and his wife, he teared up. I couldn't quite read the moment. Was he happy or upset? I went over to make sure he was okay. He grabbed my arm.

"You know why this worked?" he asked.

"Why, Roger?"

"Because it ain't cheap," he said, wiping his eyes. "It ain't cheap. That's why. Thank you for that."

I knew what Roger meant. The books were just three-ring binders. The stories and the images that inspired them were just copied in Beth's office, and the elders in the day center assembled them. We had splurged on the full-color copying of the butterfly cover, but really, the books were pretty inexpensive. But they weren't cheap. They showed thought and care. They showed an investment of time and effort. Mostly, they showed belief in the value of the elders themselves and of the stories they created together. Philosopher Susan Wolf tells us that meaning in life comes when our subjective sense of meaning meets a more objective sense of meaning.[1] In other words, meaning comes when both you and your community value the same thing. In that little celebration at the day center, with families and staff gathered together, with handmade signs and donated food, with photographic portraits and hand-copied books, we had made meaning together.

Happiness or joy can spring from immediate pleasure in the moment. Meaningfulness, on the other hand, needs more cooks and more time to cook. To practice creative care is to practice the art of meaning-making. But what exactly is meaning, and how do we create it? Is there a recipe?

Meaning in life is the subject of countless ruminations by scholars and sages alike, in disciplines from theology to philosophy, from psychology to occupational therapy. According to the American Occupational Therapy Association, occupational therapists "enable people of all ages to live life to its fullest by helping them promote health, and prevent—or live better with—injury, illness, or disability."[2] Within the field, researchers like Moses Ikiugu aim to identify which activities are meaningful, which are psychologically rewarding, and which will lead to positive feelings; a release of dopamine; and, in turn, feelings of well-being. For Ikiugu, a meaningful activity is one that one chooses for oneself, that has a goal, that connects one to others, and that is mentally stimulating.[3]

Psychologist Viktor Frankl, whose quotation opens this chapter, posits that the search for meaning is *the* central human drive, not some shadow of other instinctual drives for things like food or sex. Frankl's theories crystallized in his survival of Nazi concentration camps. He believed that finding meaning in passing moments gave him the will to survive. For Frankl, there are three routes to meaning: "(1) by creating a work or doing a deed; (2) by experiencing something or encountering someone; and (3) by the attitude we take toward unavoidable suffering."[4]

Frankl certainly saw unavoidable suffering in the death camps. Families experiencing memory loss and dementia may well face similar challenges, suffering at the hands of the cruelty of disease and sometimes at the hands of the care system itself. Creating something together and opening ourselves to connecting to others can guide us toward meaning and toward answering questions that haunt the end of life. Why did this happen? What was the purpose of my life?

My own definition of meaningfulness echoes Frankl's and arises at the crossroads where my work facilitating expression with frail elders and my work as a scholar meet. While I draw on research, over the years people like Roger have either clearly articulated a definition of meaningfulness or have lived it with me.

In 2009, as the director of the Center on Age and Community (since renamed the Center for Aging and Translational Research) at the University of Wisconsin–Milwaukee, I had the good fortune to gather together thought leaders for a think tank that I called "How to Radically Transform Activities in Long-Term Care." The heads of some of the largest US-based organizations serving older adults came together with artists who had long and deep experience using the arts for social change, many of whom had no experience working with older adults. Programming for older adults, we all agreed, wildly underestimated their capacity. What would *meaningful* programming look like? After strenuous discussion, we agreed as a group on four elements of meaningfulness. First, it invited personal expression of any form. Second, meaningfulness was pleasurable, either as an intellectual challenge or as good old-fashioned fun. Third, meaningfulness offered a sense of purpose by connecting the person to the larger world in some way. And finally, meaningfulness had value to both the elders themselves and to their larger community. It went without saying that a meaningful activity would be done by choice.

After we arrived at the four elements of meaningfulness, I asked the group to create some examples. I printed out a list of 101 activities for people with dementia from the Alzheimer's Association website, cut the list up, and handed the activities out to the small groups that blended artists, aging-services providers, and scholars. Could they "enchant" these activities? Could they apply our new elements of meaningfulness and transform "sorting silverware" or "folding napkins" into meaning-making experiences?

One of the ideas that sprang from the group of artists and aging-services professionals was inspired by an activity that one of the attendees, an activity staff member from an area day center, had actually done. At the time, the Alzheimer's Association's list of 101 recommended activities included "clipping coupons." This might sound dreadfully boring and devoid of meaning to some people, but growing up in the Midwest, I knew firsthand both the pleasure in frugality and tradition and the need that drives this deep-seated ritual.

Here is how this particular coupon-clipping activity unfolded. A group of elders gathered around a table with brightly colored newspapers and magazines. Staff invited the elders to find coupons that drew their attention and to share stories about them. What was it about the product that drew them? Did they use it? Did the product remind them of something they used? Or had they never used the product and were drawn to it by its foreignness? Whatever the reason, the facilitator invited them to share a story about the product in the coupon: Chicken pot pie? Laundry detergent? Batteries?

Together the elders carefully wrote their stories on sturdy sheets of paper and cut them with pinking shears to create an unusual border. Then the group picked a local grocery store and arranged a trip to the store in the day center van. Together, the elders boarded the van, with wheelchairs and walkers; with stories, coupons, and tape. When they got to the store, they unloaded and broke into teams, each team taking a coupon, a story, and some tape. The teams walked the aisles in search of the product featured in their coupon. When they found it, they taped the story and the coupon to the shelf and then, without a word, found their way back to the van. The elders had left anonymous gifts of story and coupons—paying it forward to unsuspecting neighbors.

What was the meaning created in this case? If, like Ikiugu, your concern is the activation of neural pathways to release dopamine, the activity was devilishly *fun*, *connected to others*, *goal-oriented*, and *mentally stimulating*. In the eyes of Frankl, the elders were creating a work and encountering others. Their attitude toward suffering was that purpose and playfulness in the moment eclipsed the various diseases or conditions they may have carried with them. In the terms of meaningfulness our group had distilled, the coupon adventure invited *self-expression* through both story and the many choices hidden in the unfolding project, from which coupon to select to which store would be the lucky recipient of their gifts. The project was both *thoughtful* and *fun*. It *connected the elders to the larger world* by leaving gifts for unknown neighbors. And the adventure *had value*; in the monetary value of the coupon, the thought put into the design, the quality of the materials, and the time and attention expended in creating the stories.

The artists and aging-services professionals gathered for the think tank enchanted a good half-dozen activities. "Sorting silverware" became a virtual dinner party held in two day centers, one in Milwaukee and one in Detroit. Elders would choose a menu reflecting their own cultural backgrounds, choose the decorations, design the invitations, participate in the meal creation, and welcome their guests via Skype. "String up Cheerios for birds" evolved into a multiphase project that involved learning about area birds, drawing the birds, naming them, inviting the elders to share memories of birds, creating new stories about them, inviting people to the event, and finally stringing up the Cheerios and presenting them as a gift to the birds at the onset of winter. The activity created meaning in that it offered fun and pleasure, an opportunity for personal expression, and a way to connect to the larger world with rigor and value.

The invitation to enchant daily activities is embedded in TimeSlips' Creative Care Institute, where artists and caregivers, both professional and personal, gather to learn engagement- and community-building techniques. Ideas for meaningful projects that have emerged from the institute over the years have truly astonished me. One group at a training in Tempe, Arizona, transformed "feed the ducks" into a full-scale, citywide, cross-generational Festival of the Duck. And yet these simple guidelines can also be applied at the other end of the scale, to quiet moments in one's living room. One woman shared that she had created a game out of folding laundry. She invited her husband to help her fold sheets. With each fold they would move closer together until, with the final fold, they would embrace. At one training, a young woman shared a story about visiting with an older neighbor, a woman who lived alone and who had some significant cognitive challenges. Every month the neighbor received a "fruit of the month" package from her daughter, who lived far away. Together, the young woman and her neighbor stumbled upon a meaningful way to thank the neighbor's daughter. They held the fruit, smelled it, and observed it closely. Then they took the postcard that came inside the box and, on the back of the card, wrote down several words describing the fruit. Then they mailed the poem back to the daughter: a gift in return for her gift.

Research in positive psychology tells us that altruism makes people feel good. Volunteering, sharing expertise with others, doing small acts of kindness for others—all these contribute to our well-being. But too often those who are frail or disabled are imagined as incapable of giving. Too often the care relationship is imagined as one empty vessel, the older person, and one full vessel, the caregiver. In this strange and all-too-prevalent concept of care, caregivers pour themselves into the empty vessel until they themselves are empty. This mistaken concept of care ignores the capacity and need for those who receive care to connect to the world beyond them and to give back.

Aging and frailty push us inward. Loss of friends and family push us toward living with memories of people rather than forging new connections. The stigma of aging, of dementia, and of loneliness can create a force field that people bump up against and walk away from. So do guilt and the awkwardness of not knowing how to connect. To practice creative care is to move through the force field to invite someone into a meaning-making process. The person might say no. Saying no should always be a choice. But the invitation should include a turn outward toward the larger community and a consideration of what gift could be shared with the world. It might be a coupon and a story of the smell of laundry detergent. It might be a string of Cheerios shared with a sparrow named Stan who sticks out the winter. It might be a three-word poem about cantaloupe. It might be a multiday, citywide Festival of the Duck. Whatever it is, the gift shouldn't be "cheap." It should resonate with what Roger felt in that simplest of celebrations, with three-ring binders of stories being shared with families and storytellers. It should ring with the feeling that Roger's words, and Roger himself, matter.

✦

Connecting to the
Larger World from Home

This part of the book is already full of examples that caregivers can easily try at home. But perhaps the first step is to take an inventory of assets. I don't mean one's worldly goods, but rather skills and small things that you might be able to use to connect to others.

Do you have perennials in your yard from which you might share cuttings or flowers?

Care partners might work together to share these with a neighbor or a nearby shelter or care home.

Can your loved one living with dementia read aloud from books?

Care partners might arrange to volunteer to read to children.

Does either the person with dementia or the caregiver play an instrument?

Together, you might try setting a story or a poem to music, recording it, and sending it to family or friends. Or singing a well-known song together and recording and sharing it. Smartphones are miraculous tools for this.

Do either of you have favorite meals and recipes?

Together, you might prepare recipes, photograph the results, and write them up and share with family as your own family cookbook.

Can the person with dementia write cursive? Read cursive? Tie a tie?

Caregivers might arrange sharing that skill with grandchildren or neighboring kids.

Do you or your care partner have lots of old costume jewelry?

There are a growing number of organizations that transform or "up-cycle" costume jewelry into new creations.

If you visit and enjoy creative storytelling on the TimeSlips website at www.timeslips.org and want to share this with others, you might host an Engagement Party or a story session at a local library.

Engagement Parties are informal gatherings of friends and family designed to teach simple creative engagement techniques. All information about hosting an Engagement Party can be found on www .timeslips.org.

Do you or your care partner have broken things in your garage that you might take apart and transform into a museum with stories attached to different items?

Invite neighbors to take the items and stories.

Do you or your care partner have a supply of old stationery or postcards that you might send to people?

Faith-based communities or area agencies on aging often have lists of people who could use some cheering up.

These ideas invite you to look at your belongings and skills with fresh eyes. They also ask you to let go of any shame or hesitancy to reach out and connect with neighbors, family, and friends. You will be doing them a favor by letting them know that dementia is a part of life—and that people with dementia or other frailties in late life can be loving and caring.

CHAPTER 8

Opening Yourself to Wonder

To wonder is now ever so quickly followed by knowing, and too often the stamping out of the opportunity for a good that arises in the face of uncertainty or the sublime.

LAWRENCE WESCHLER,
Introduction to *Wonder*

It is not understanding that destroys wonder, it is familiarity.

JOHN STUART MILL,
An Examination of Sir William
Hamilton's Philosophy

"I wonder . . ." we say when we are teasing out the possibilities of something we are uncertain about. Thinkers from Aristotle to St. Thomas Aquinas have defined wonder as a positive drive toward curiosity, toward pursuing the answer to an idea or a mystery. To be in a state of wonder is to suddenly walk smack into the limits of your knowledge and to be inspired to push beyond them by questioning, learning, and growing.

In creative care, wonder is found in the contradiction between a dire diagnosis and a smile that widens a person's face in raw joy. Wonder can be found when people whose charts declare their reduced capacity reveal unexpected and marvelous strengths: Telling a joke. Creating a poignant metaphor. Drawing an arm across the body with an elegance that stops you cold in its delicate beauty. In creative care, wonder walks us to the brink of one of the hardest questions of all, asked by so many grieving children and spouses, friends and loved ones: "Does he remember me?" "Does she know who I am?"

But wonder is also the answer to those questions. Wonder invites us to suspend what we think we know about personality patterns, brain scans, and stages of disease. It invites us into a state of curiosity in which we can assume that meaningful expression and connection are possible. In more than twenty years of working with people with profound cognitive challenges, I have experienced hundreds of moments when I was "gobsmacked" (as Lawrence Weschler so colorfully writes in his introduction to the book *Wonder*) by an unexpected response, or a moment of powerful emotional connection. Weschler describes the breathtaking moment of wonder when "one notices how, in astonishment, a pillow of air has formed and become lodged in one's very mouth and that one has neither breathed in nor out for what seems a good ten-second eternity."[1] In some ways, all the stories in this book reflect these unexpected "pillow of air" moments. But I share three specific moments here in hopes of relaying the rewards of holding oneself in an open, suspended sense of wonder.

The first is a story that pioneering and visionary choreographer Liz Lerman shared with me, and later published in her book of essays, *Hiking the Horizontal*. Liz's uncle was at the end of his life. Her family gathered at the hospital to comfort her aunt, who was distraught. Her uncle was in a coma, and as they gathered together in his hospital room waiting for the end, his arms were spasming rather violently. Liz's aunt begged the staff to sedate him to calm the jerky movements. But that would certainly mean the end of any possibility that he could connect with them before he passed. Liz asked her aunt for permission to try something. What would it be like, she wondered, to move *with* him? What would his movements, at this profound moment in his life, feel like? Were they only meaningless spasms? Or was there more to them? Liz's aunt agreed to the experiment, so Liz took her uncle's hands into hers and let his movements lead her. "I just followed wherever his arms took me. It didn't feel as jerky as it looked. It didn't seem to be about nervousness at all, more of a kind of gliding through the air," she wrote. Watching this shared moment, Liz's aunt asked if she could try it. And so his final moments shifted, from sedation to expression. "The last image I have of my uncle alive is seeing my aunt dancing with him," wrote Lerman. They did this for the last two days of his life. Was he aware? They couldn't know. But opening themselves to the wonder of the moment created an opportunity for connection and meaning.[2]

More than 150 people were seated at training tables stuffed into the chapel of a long-term-care community in St. Paul, Minnesota. I was there to offer a half-day training workshop in creative story-telling. The host site arranged for me to do a live demonstration of creative storytelling with a group of elders with dementia whom the staff had gathered in a common room of their nursing home, and live-streamed it back down to the training room. The storytellers were a little slow to jump into the process at first, which was under-standable considering it was the very first time they had met or engaged with me. But after a few minutes, the group caught the rhythm of the storytelling and shared some lovely answers. The session was filled with laughter and slow but certain smiles. When I came back down to the training room and opened the floor to questions, one woman asked, "How do you select the people to participate?" Before I could answer, the staff member who had helped arrange the demonstration session jumped in.

"Can I answer that?"

"Of course," I remember saying.

"Draw the names from a hat," she said.

She explained that she had deliberately selected people whom she thought couldn't actually participate. Watching them open to this and respond, she was ashamed that she had assumed they couldn't do it. "So that's my suggestion," she said again, "draw the names out of a hat." One just never knows who will open up to the invitation to imagine. Even now, with years of experience in facilitating creative engagement, sometimes I feel like the most valuable thing I bring with me when I walk into a care setting is my complete lack of knowledge of people's various diagnoses, their lists of pills and treatment plans, and any sense of the limitations that form under the daily weight of reduced expectations. I simply bring wonder.

A story from a recent TimeSlips session at a day center in the heart of Milwaukee also captures both sides of wonder, meeting the limits of our knowledge and moving past them with curiosity. Mr. Wilson was quiet. His eyes were tracking us as we moved around the room, but there was a vagueness behind them. He had a distinguished air, with more salt than pepper in his hair, and a solidity to the set of his shoulders. He was a regular at the Milwaukee day center where Elaine, one of our master trainers, was working with staff to offer regular TimeSlips sessions on Tuesday afternoons. What was he understanding? Could he hear? Did he recognize Elaine, who came each week? Or Sheila, the staff member who welcomed him every day? When we finished welcoming the small group of elders to the session, Elaine posed her beautiful question to start the creative journey that would sweep us away for the next hour. Or so we hoped.

"Can you teach us a game you played in childhood?" she asked the group, using her outside voice.

The phrasing was complex. People looked understandably puzzled as the question seeped in.

Sheila jumped in and rephrased.

"Think about games you played when you were a kid. Is there one you could teach us?"

Elaine has been working with this group for nearly a year, training Sheila as a facilitator. I admire how well they work together, how well they know the elders, how well the two of them can sense when the group needs more explanation or encouragement.

The magic starts slowly. One woman says, "Swimming."

"Can you show us how?" asks Elaine, modeling some arm movements that might be but aren't quite swimming, leaving room for the storyteller to define the movements herself.

And that she does, stretching her arms forward into a crawl and then backward. It was an impressive range of movement. Then she pitched forward, hands together, into a dive. Sheila ran over to keep her from landing on the floor.

"Whoa!" said Elaine. The group joined her laughter. "It's the shallow end—let's not dive too deep!"

One gentleman drew a circle with his cane and pitched imaginary marbles.

One instructed the group in a game of duck duck goose, making Sheila and Elaine run around the circle of chairs and wheelchairs.

Pearl, a tiny woman in a wheelchair, had a bright light behind her eyes.

"Swing," she said in a mischievous voice, when Elaine asked her what game she would teach us.

"How could you show that?"

Pearl pulled her arms slowly back and then slowly forward, then again, back and forward rhythmically. It was subtle, but we could feel the swing. The whole group jumped in, pulling arms back slowly and forward again, back and forth, back and forth, together in rhythm.

"Higher," whispered one of the facilitators playfully.

And we did. As arms pumped a little further back and a little further forward, a sound rose from the group that could only be described as a communal "Weeeeeeee!" with each forward arm movement.

We were swinging.

Then we turned to Mr. Wilson.

"What do you think, Mr. Wilson?" said Elaine. "What game would you like to teach us?"

He stared at her for a moment, as though absorbing the question, as though drawing on her focus to focus himself. I wasn't sure whether he would answer, or whether he understood the question. Elaine and Sheila paused. And waited.

Then he put out his hand and slowly moved it up and down as though bouncing a ball. He picked up the imaginary ball and made a perfect jump shot to Bruce, a facilitator on the other side of the room. Bruce caught the imaginary ball. He bounced it and shot it back to Mr. Wilson, who caught it, bounced it, and shot it back to Bruce. And again. And again. For five minutes. The rest of the group reviewed the games and replayed the games. But Mr. Wilson and Bruce kept passing and shooting baskets.

Does he even know who I am?

To open oneself to wonder, conceding the limits of our knowledge, is to admit that we don't know the answer to that question. We can't know. Moments of lucidity can flash in unexpected moments. Mr. Wilson might not have answered. Or he might have made an imaginary three-pointer off Bruce's rebound pass. We can't know which way a moment will fork. More crucially perhaps, if we consider identity to be relational, if we do not treat someone as if they are fully human and capable of meaningful response, we ourselves are not fully human. To enact our humanity, we create conditions in which others can express their own. When Bruce caught the three-pointer and tossed it back to Mr. Wilson, he not only said, "Yes, and," but he also opened himself to the wonder of the moment. Led by his curiosity, he tried some variations. He bounce-passed the imaginary ball to Mr. Wilson, who caught it, and bounce-passed it back. He dribbled it between his legs and tossed it back. Led by curiosity, together they played with all that an imaginary basketball could do in this moment. Will Mr. Wilson remember the moment? We can't know. But Elaine, Sheila, Bruce, and I know that we will and, holding that memory for him, we can invite him back to that moment again and again.

Open Yourself to Wonder at Home

Wonder falls into two camps. The first contains things that are simply unknowable and that we have to find peace with. They include questions like these:

Will this disease or aging process go quickly? Slowly?
How much time do we have left?
Is there something we could have done differently to avoid this?
Will it happen to me?
Why?

To open yourself to wonder with these questions is to acknowledge they are unknowable.

Try writing down the question or questions that haunt you on a beautiful piece of paper. Take care to write them clearly, in your best handwriting. Put the paper in an envelope with no stamp or address and drop it in the mailbox. Say goodbye to the envelope and question as you do.

The second camp of wonder contains things about which we can be curious and let that curiosity ignite our interest and give direction and energy to the moments of our days together. Here are some beautiful questions you can use to spark wonder in daily moments:

Whatever happened to . . . ?

Where did this come from?

What happens if I turn this upside down?

What if I do this backwards?

What if I do this faster? Or slower?

What if I made this much bigger? Or much smaller?

Artists know these kinds of questions well. They fuel the creative process.

CHAPTER 9

All of the Above— Cultivating Awe in Our Lives

When I was about ten, my parents packed my brother and me into my dad's tiny car and drove us out of southern Wisconsin's flat expanses of rich, black topsoil to the piney crags of Colorado. This was my first encounter with mountains, and my first memory of *awe*. Hugging a curve in the little green car, we'd open suddenly to a vast expanse of sky, rock, trees, valley, and water in various formations that took one's breath away. My mom developed a phrase for this experience. "Look! A magnificent vista!" she would exclaim. That quickly became a catchphrase for all of us. We would point out magnificent vistas all across Wyoming and Montana. As we returned back to the flatlands of the Midwest, I learned to find awe in the subtle rise of the horizon in the gentle rolling cornfields. "Look! A magnificent vista!" I say it today with my own kids. Crossing the St. Croix river into Minneapolis. Sitting on the dock at my parents' cabin, watching the fuchsia summer sunsets. Even just looking out our living-room window in fall at the sweep of oranges and reds on the maples lining the yard: what a magnificent vista.

"Awesome," people say now, almost as often as earlier generations said "cool." Splashed about so cavalierly, awe is in danger of losing its power as a word. A deeper understanding of awe's qualities is worth safeguarding. Awe, I believe, can be a guiding principle of how to live and how to invite others into meaningful relationship with the world. Awe can be a gateway to meaningfulness. The feeling of awe has two parts: a sensation of vastness and a challenge to our frame of reference. In the most rudimentary sense, awe is having one's mind blown. The field of study around awe is just emerging. We have much to understand, particularly about differences between negative experiences of awe, like hurricanes or other large-scale tragic events, and positive experiences of awe. Current studies suggest that experiencing positive sensations of awe can decrease stress and inflammation[1] and increase one's well-being.[2] When we feel small in the face of something bigger than ourselves, that increases our sense of shared humanity. One emerges from the moment more humble and kinder to others—perhaps seeing our fellow small and fragile humans in a new, shared light.[3] Paul Piff's 2015 study found that "a small dose of awe even gave participants a momentary boost in life satisfaction," a finding that underscores "the importance and promise of cultivating awe in everyday life."[4]

We commonly experience awe in one of three ways: through nature, through spiritual practice, or through art in all of its manifestations. We can feel swept up by the power of a symphony or the energy pulsing through a live concert. Singing in a choir provides an immediate feeling of vastness in the combination and capacity of human voices brought together as one. In our early days of dating, my husband and I would visit the Museum of Modern Art and sit in front of a Jackson Pollock painting, tipping upside down on the bench in front of the painting in order to fall into the dynamic world of the canvas.

Those many and early moments of "magnificent vistas" were addictive for me. I found myself in the mountains of Colorado for college. Back home in the Midwest now for many years, I make a pilgrimage to the vast horizon of Lake Michigan nearly every day. There is something incredibly calming about that endless horizon line, its colors, moods, and power changing nearly every day with complete disregard for whatever is troubling me. For a moment, when I turn the corner and run down the path curving toward the lake, my list of things to do disappears and my worries shrink. Sometimes they even stay shrunk. Awe has a way of reordering, prioritizing, and calming in a heartbeat. I become what researchers call a "small self" in the face of vastness—of space, time, and ideas.

After twenty-five years of facilitating creative engagement with elders, I have come to believe that there is a fourth portal to awe. In addition to nature, spiritual beliefs, and art or creativity, one can access awe by connecting to the vastness of another human soul. Some might equate this with spiritual belief. In fact, some use the framework of spiritual practice to contain all elements of awe, considering nature and art as access points to spirituality. But my goal here is to identify concrete ways we can experience awe in our daily lives and to facilitate the experience of awe for others. That work is built on opening oneself to recognizing and engaging deeply with other people's humanity.

The pillars of creative care outlined in earlier chapters—living "Yes, and"; asking beautiful questions; offering proof of listening; connecting to the larger world; opening oneself to wonder—all accumulate to an experience of awe.

One of my most powerful experiences of awe happened at the confluence of nature, art, and deep connection with another human being, a man named Jim. Jim was hard to reach. He had lost all verbal language. I myself wasn't sure whether Jim was reachable, and my uncertainty led to both my feeling of vastness in the beauty he created and a reorganization of my thinking about the capacities of people with cognitive disabilities. I share Jim's story here as a way to demonstrate awe in action. The story is drawn from a blend of memory and video recordings, and then checked and approved by Jim's wife, Fran, herself.

It was a gray, winter day in 2013. Five of us were crowded into the tiny kitchen of a lower duplex apartment on Milwaukee's East Side: me; the owners, Jim and his wife, Fran; their caregiver, Ann; and their care manager, Katie. Five of us stood around the table with a cat weaving among our ten legs. There were two chairs, but midwestern politeness prohibited us from using them. Fran offered us tea from a pan on the stove. It smelled of chamomile and lavender.

In the moment, they looked to me to start the conversation.

"I'm just here to introduce myself and learn from you," I said, hoping to divert the focus from me back to the group. "I'm part of a project called the Islands of Milwaukee. We're learning how to bring creativity to folks living at home, alone or underconnected to community."

The project team had worked hard for that language. In focus group after focus group, we pushed words like "lonely," "isolated," and "homebound" out of our vocabulary in favor of words in which the people described could actually recognize themselves. "Under-connected"—weren't we all at least a little underconnected?

Jim was a formidable and animated presence: tall and lean, his green, oiled-canvas hat tilted up slightly at the brim. He was clearly watching the room but would not meet my eyes. He had the look of having just come in from a long hike, and his muscles vibrated with the desire to launch themselves on another. He would take a step forward and then back. Forward, sideways, back. In his mid-seventies, his dementia had taken his ability to speak, but he engaged with the world fully, through movement. Fran had to hire a caregiver to start walking with him when she couldn't keep up with his ten-mile-a-day pace. He had been a university instructor in environmental philosophy and was deeply connected—physically, spiritually, psychologically—to nature.

Open yourself to wonder. Curiosity is a sign of respect.

I looked around the room. On the kitchen table was a small cutting board, a plastic red paring knife, and broccoli and red peppers cut into tiny pieces and arranged into clusters.

"Jim loves to cut and arrange things. In colors, patterns. I see him as an artist," said Fran.

On top of a trunk next to the stove sat at least ten pieces of driftwood, clearly selected and arranged with care.

"Jim loves to walk along the beach," said Fran. "He picks up pieces of wood. He will show them to me, and we name them. This one is 'cat.'"

Sure enough, I could make out the eyes, nose, and ears of a cat on the bulb at the end of the short piece of wood.

"And this one is 'whale,'" said Fran, and the soft arch of the driftwood took shape.

Yes, and—observe, accept, and add something positive.

"I have a question," I said. "Jim, I know you love walking along the lake. Could you show me—how does water move?"

Ask a beautiful question.

I could feel the whole room pause. Was this answerable? The right question can open a door to a shared world between people. But the wrong question can lock it tightly. I tried rephrasing.

"How does water move? Can you show me?"

Jim took a few steps over to the trunk topped with driftwood and selected a piece. He rubbed it rhythmically with his hand, which was missing two fingers above the knuckle. Slowly, he stretched his arm out to the side, the driftwood reaching across the room. He held it there, in stillness, for what seemed minutes. *Was this it?* I wondered. *Should I interrupt? Ask another question?*

Don't be afraid of stillness, silence.

Then slowly, Jim began to move his arm, leading with the driftwood. He was dancing. I looked to Fran and mouthed, "Can I film this?" and she nodded, her eyes and face again wide in wonder. I took out my phone and pressed "record." All four of us stepped backward in the cramped kitchen to find a place by the wall to give Jim as wide a berth as possible for his answer.

As he held the piece of wood aloft, in his hands it became buoyant, in sync with the movement of waves that he supplied with his arms. The piece of wood took a slow journey across calm but capricious waters, moving from relative stillness to a slow rolling toward the shore. When that piece of driftwood completed its journey, Jim arranged it on the trunk by the stove and picked up a new piece—introduced it to us, rubbed it as though both cleansing it and bringing out its inner beauty—and then that piece could begin its own unique dance across the water.

Open yourself to wonder.

What did it mean? Did an answer matter? Jim's grace and strength were breathtaking. He would slowly transfer his energy from one extended arm to the other, shifting his weight from left foot to right, from right back to left. Suddenly, he was not "disabled." We weren't gathered into this tiny kitchen for a care crisis. He was a master puppeteer, a dancer, an artist. His audience of four stared with mouths open and eyes wide for nearly twenty minutes as he animated each piece of wood on its own unique journey across the waves.

When he placed the last piece of driftwood back on the trunk, the room took a collective exhale.

"That was just beautiful, Jim. Thank you so much for that gift," I said.

He continued to stare beyond us all.

Connect to the larger world.

"I would like to share this with some artists, is that okay?" I asked.

Jim's eyes locked on something beyond me.

"Oh yes—please do," said Fran.

Months later, I returned to the tiny kitchen, this time with two artists who had watched the video of Jim's dance and developed their own interpretation of it. Jim had moved into a nearby care community and was adjusting to his new life, as was Fran, who was finally able to sleep. When I asked whether she wanted to see what the performers had created, she was enthusiastic and asked if they could show it to her in the garden out back—the garden that Jim had planted and tended for so many years.

It was one of those fall days in the Midwest that takes your breath away. Warm yellow light with long shadows that fills you with gratitude for the chance to wear short sleeves one last time that season. James Hart and Rebecca Martinez, two artists with Sojourn Theatre, each carried a piece of driftwood into the garden and found a place. Katie and Anne—the caregivers who had been with us on that day months earlier—were seated next to me; and two guests, the Sojourn Theatre director Maureen Towey and artist Liz Lerman, who happened to be visiting, filled out the audience.

I found myself watching Fran watching the movements that so clearly echoed the long-limbed dance of her beloved. "Oh, oh. Oh, oh," she said in quiet exhales throughout. "Oh, oh. Oh, oh." When they finished the brief performance, I asked Fran if she wanted to guide them to any changes, or if she might want to join them. She wasn't sure at first, but when they began again, Fran stood up and joined them, echoing their echoes of Jim's offering.

We had taken a video and still photos that she could show Jim and that we would include in an art exhibit in Milwaukee's City Hall. I asked Fran if she wanted to give the dance a name. She thought for a moment.

"Dance for the Love of Jim," she said.

Several years later I sat down with Fran outside her church, on a fall day reminiscent of that day in the garden. My experience with Jim had a profound effect on me, and I wanted to hear the story from her perspective. I wanted to understand the why and how of those deep connections. At the time, Jim was still living several blocks away at the Milwaukee Catholic Home, and Fran visited often, accompanied by family and friends from church.

"What happened that day . . . he responded to something in you, and he didn't know you," Fran said. "I mean because of who you are and the work you are doing, he opened up in ways I've never seen him. We've been married fifty-three years, and I've never seen anything like what he did that day."

She paused, took a moment, and then continued: "Your presence could be described as deep listening. And that's what I think Jim— that there is a certain thing that can happen to him even now, and it happens if he has that sense. I can see it in his face. If he has that sense that someone is really, really listening, it's like he is, on some level, that he is right there with you."

Offer proof of listening.

"Even in silence," said Fran. "You can do that even when no one is saying anything at all."

Just after I realized that Mom was beginning to experience dementia, a friend who knew I was writing this book encouraged me to invite Mom to write with me. She said she was game but preferred that I ask her questions by email so she could think about them. So it happened that one day I emailed her about awe.

"What is awe, and when do you feel it?" I wrote.

She responded quickly—this time, with none of the usual trouble of pausing and getting the answer lost in her draft folder:

> Awe comes when something wonderful or unexpected comes to a person. It could be when you are seeing your newborn baby or grandchild; seeing how tall Ben *[my older son]* became last year; how kind someone is to you and takes care of you, like Dad does for me. It could be during

a spectacular event in nature, like a beautiful sunrise or sunset or seeing the beauty of the Catalina mountains when I get up in the morning. I was in awe of Henry *[my nephew]* when I saw his routine in *Hamilton*, of Will's *[my younger son]* smile when he sees you. I can even be in awe of finding a perfect jacket or dress like my new red one.

I had emailed only Mom, but Dad wrote back, too—Dad the atheist, suspicious of anything that smells of religion; yet also Dad the guy who made sure his kids understood the power and beauty of nature, and who cries in musicals and when he reads a good poem.

Hmmmm. Awe? Not a word I often use, but as I think about it, a word that does describe how I occasionally feel. It is how I felt when I was sitting in my car and you called to tell us about the MacArthur. It is how I feel when nature belittles us with a hurricane, or a tornado or massive brush fires. Being in awe of something doesn't always mean something beautiful, it can be horrifying. So I guess I am in awe of nature's natural forces, their unpredictability, sometimes good and sometimes not so good. Like being in awe of a beautiful snowfall on a cold winter's night.

Or, perhaps, the hurricane of emotions in the experience of caring for someone with dementia.

Does the impulse to altruism the researchers found in experiences of awe hold if the awe is inspired by the vastness of something tragic?

The stories of everyday heroes were nearly endless in the coverage of hurricane-stricken Houston, Florida, and Puerto Rico. The heroics of everyday caregivers still go largely unnoticed. I can imagine a photograph: It is several years from now. Dad is helping Mom put on her favorite red jacket. I look on with relief and gratitude for the vastness of his capacity to care, mind blown.

Awe brings us together into a shared moment that connects us in the face of something vast and inspires us to rethink what we thought we knew. Awe directs us toward meaningfulness by compelling humility and belonging, as well as individual learning and growth triggered through wonder. We can use the elements of creative care to invite another person into a shared experience of awe—transforming our relationships, our lives. We can also use these same elements to invite entire communities and systems of care into a shared experience of awe—transforming the way we provide care itself and the way communities relate to elders, people with disabilities, and their care partners. In the next part of the book I turn toward stories of what I learned from participating in or observing expansive community-building projects that have done just that, with the potential to infuse meaning into daily moments with people we love and care for. This is the great hope: that if enough people learn the techniques, creative care might be poured like water into care systems themselves and change the way we understand and deliver care.

✦

Cultivating Moments
of Awe at Home

Awe is an experience of vastness that invites us to reconsider what we know and understand. It can be triggered by connections to nature, creativity or art, spirituality, and other people.

A first step toward cultivating moments of awe at home is simply to ask yourself, family, and friends, "What fills you with awe?" Keep a list and use it to guide your practice of cultivating awe. The most common answers I hear are these:

- Sunset

- Sunrise

- A sudden thunderstorm

- Babies

- Grandchildren

- Beautiful music

It might not be possible to experience these directly. Sometimes it's tough to be awake and ready for sunrise or sunset, for example. But you might try to access these experiences through art.

1. Draw a sunset (or sunrise), and invite and write down words that express our feelings about that.

2. Imagine being in a thunderstorm. Make the sounds you would hear in a thunderstorm. Share a story of any memories of being in a storm.

3. Create a page for each grandchild. Put a photo or a simple drawing of the grandchild in the center. Add descriptive words of what you know about the grandchild around the photo. Add your hopes and wishes to the page. Put the pages in a folder where you can add to them and review them together.

4. Simply listen to beautiful music together. Or invite friends or family to listen with you. You might identify several songs that you can sing together or join (or start!) a choir.

Artists also know that playing with both a sense of expectation and scale can create feelings of awe. The WONDER exhibit at the Renwick Gallery in Washington, DC, featured a room filled with piles and piles of buttons—thousands upon thousands of buttons. Another room was filled with a huge tree crafted in segments and suspended in the air on its side. Another featured thousands of bugs arranged as wallpaper decoration. These questions might help inspire you:

• What if you gathered and arranged a thousand of some everyday object—paper clips, stones?

• What if you made a tiny model of something that is normally large?

- What if you made an everyday object special and unexpected?

- What if you went somewhere where you feel small—among trees, maybe, or at a vast beach?

- What if you went somewhere where you felt very big— watching a colony of ants, perhaps?

PART THREE

Changing Care Through Creativity

CHAPTER 10

Penelope, the Hero Who Never Left Home

The magic of the moment when I showed a group a picture of the Marlboro Man in order to create a story happened on a long-ago spring day in 1996. After that moment, I single-mindedly tried to re-create that moment for years. And years. In setting after setting. In day centers and nursing homes. In private homes and apartment buildings. In senior centers and even libraries and art museums. Time after time, the magic came back. In this part of the book, I explore how, compelled by that magic, I tried to take the principles covered in part 2 to see whether they could be applied on a larger scale to change the very way we understand, practice, and provide care.

I quickly turned to modeling the approach and teaching caregivers that connection flourishes when we shift away from the expectation of memory and toward the freedom of imagination and shared expression. The people I trained in turn trained others: family members, students, volunteers, professionals at every level. Together we would discover that meaning emerges when we build a shared world by inviting and echoing creative responses to a prompt—be it an image, an object, a song, or a question.

I formed a limited liability corporation (LLC) and then a nonprofit called TimeSlips to bring the approach to as many people as we could. TimeSlips staff worked with researchers to test the impact of the approach, finding significant benefits.[1] For years, TimeSlips trainers coached people to take the stories that emerged from those sessions and share them with others—to connect to the larger world and to use the creative output to help change how people thought about late life in general and about dementia in particular. In some cases, the TimeSlips team created art exhibits and plays in well-known museums and theaters.

But then I started wondering: *What if...*

Could we go further? TimeSlips was commonly considered a "therapy," operating within the medical framework. TimeSlips was an "intervention" to improve "patients." Was there unique power in *not* being medicine? Were we missing out on the community-building power of the arts?

My wondering intensified and began to shape a new project. What if the elders really had an opportunity to dive deeply into a large-scale creative project, as artists do when they tackle creating a new piece of theater, a novel, a film, or an original score? What if the entire community of care, staff, elders, and volunteers, could be invited into this project as one enormous ensemble? What if this project was so interesting that families actually wanted to leave work early once a week to join their mom or dad in the workshop session in the independent apartments, day center, assisted living, or skilled nursing home? What if the project was so interesting and so infused into the daily life of the organization that staff at all levels not only knew about the project but also felt welcome to participate? What if the culminating project was a professionally produced play, staged inside the care home, and featuring anyone from the care community who wanted to perform?

What if care settings truly became places of culture and meaning-making?

These questions fed the dream that became the Penelope project. The idea began in 2009, when I asked Beth Meyer Arnold, my friend who ran Adult Day Services at Luther Manor, if she would be open to a project that reimagined Homer's *Odyssey* from the perspective of his wife and queen, Penelope. We would take apart the story and create an original play that we would stage, professionally, inside the nursing home. Beth stared at me. "I don't know what you're talking about, but yes," she said. We'd been collaborating for more than fifteen years at that point. We both trusted our hunches. And our hunch was that, although this huge idea seemed impossible, we would find a way to make the project happen.

The artistic collaboration with Sojourn Theatre came from a stroke of good timing. Over coffee with my old friend Michael Rohd, he asked me what projects I was working on. I told him I had this crazy idea to do a professionally produced play in collaboration with a long-term care community. The problem was, I didn't have a theater company. Well, he did. And it was a good one that specialized in site-specific performances tackling social issues. And so the partnership with Sojourn Theatre was forged.

I described the project to my university theater department at one of our monthly meetings. They didn't understand how it could benefit students to put on a play in a nursing home. Would they learn to hang lights? To run a soundboard? Clearly not. But my department chair found a way to support it financially, and my colleague Robin Mello and I integrated the project into several classes—two that would help us gather input to shape the play, and one that would support the play performance itself with student actors and production crew.

Together as one giant ensemble—artists, staff, elders, students, family members, and volunteers—we would create something new that had value and that nurtured all of us. Together we would forge an entire community built on creative care.

So many stories unfolded over those two years as we all tried to do something that seemed both impossible and without a road map. The artists had created beautiful theater in nontraditional settings before, but they had never tried staging a performance in a place where people lived and where strict regulations governed nearly every aspect of daily life. Beth Meyer Arnold had established person-centered care practices in Luther Manor's day center, but staff in other areas of care still directed large group programs with little input from the elders. And none of the four areas of care had ever collaborated on a joint project before. In surveys we gave students before the project started, the majority shared that they had little to no contact with elders in their lives. Some were afraid of being in their company. A few students actively disliked older people. "I'm a waitress," I remember one student saying. "I've never had a good encounter with an older person." I'd written and produced plays inspired by TimeSlips stories before, but never staged one in situ, with the very same people who created the stories.

We were all in new territory. In the end, we created something astonishing. We created something that none of us could have imagined alone and that was only possible by giving up control and constantly opening ourselves up to one another with "Yes, and." Here are just a few stories of the growth that happened through Penelope that capture the perspective and impact of the project, as well as the range of those involved: the artists, the elders, the staff, and the students.

The Kids Are Alright

Jake was nineteen, with dusty brown hair and a sturdy build. A quiet student of architecture, he came to the storytelling class to satisfy a requirement. The class is known as a fun, easy three credits. Jake had no idea that this particular semester, the storytelling class would mostly be meeting at a long-term-care home, facilitating story workshops about Homer's *Odyssey*. None of the twenty-five students who showed up on the first day of class knew. Some dropped the class when they found out, but most stuck with it. Jake was one of them, although he didn't say more than absolutely necessary in class. I couldn't read his silence. He could be in a slow boil of frustration that could lead to him dropping the class, or he could just be shy. He had a neutral expression like a force field that made him tough to read. To prep the students for getting ready to work with older adults, my co-instructor Robin Mello and I invited Beth Meyer Arnold from Luther Manor to talk about what students could expect. What might be the range of abilities and challenges students would encounter?

What is it like to talk with someone with dementia? With someone who had experienced a stroke?

Warming up the class, Robin started with a storytelling exercise she had honed over years of teaching. "Line up in order of age," she instructed the group. When they managed to do that, she had them form a circle. So Jake, who discovered that he was the youngest person in the room, stood next to Beth, who found herself the oldest. Robin asked the youngest person to tell the group something the person had figured out about life, his own or in general, and then to ask the next person in line a question about something the person hadn't figured out yet. The statements ranged from college-student silliness to the unexpectedly poignant: From "I've figured out that if I drink six beers, I will throw up," to "I've figured out that I should call my mom at least once a week." From "I wonder if you ever stop feeling awkward at parties," to "I wonder if I'll ever stop feeling awkward in this class." By the time we got to the end, Beth, the oldest, was set to ask a question of Jake, the youngest. "How does my college-age son want to be parented? I want to be helpful and guide him but don't want to get in his way," she asked. Jake thought for a second and said, "I think you should ask him exactly what you just asked me."

Jake's going to be okay, I thought. As the semester progressed, we divided the class into four teams to work in the four areas of care at Luther Manor. Jake's group was assigned to the skilled nursing unit, where those with the most profound disabilities lived. Luther Manor is like a small village sprawling out across a million square feet, with seven hundred residents, including those attending the day center, and seven hundred staff working various shifts. Students were facilitating workshops in the independent-living, assisted-living, skilled nursing, and day center areas of the community. So Robin and I raced across the campus to try to observe each group for at least part of the class time before hopping back in the van and returning to the university.

Jake was in charge of the session in the nursing home the day I observed their group. Jean, the activity specialist, had gathered about a dozen residents into a circle, and Jake stood in the middle with a skein of rose-colored yarn. All the students wore name tags, but Jake and the others walked around the circle and introduced themselves to warm up the room before they started their activity.

"So," said Jake a little sheepishly, "The story of Penelope is basically a love story." Jake shared how moved he was by Penelope's faithfulness to Odysseus for twenty years, ten years as he fought in the war and another ten years as he wandered the sea with no word from him, and by how she raised their son by herself. "It's an important story to me right now, because I just asked my girlfriend to marry me. And she said yes."

The staff and elders cheered and congratulated him.

"But here's the thing," he added quickly, interrupting their well-wishes. "I don't have any idea what I'm doing! I'm only nineteen years old. You guys have so much more experience with love than I do. I'm hoping that you can share some stories about what you've learned about love." For every story someone told, they got to hold a piece of the rose yarn. Then as the next story unfolded, the students extended the yarn to them. By the end of the thirty-minute session, the room was crisscrossed in a chaotic cat's cradle and full of stories of love. There was the love of parents. Of children. Of a pet parakeet. Of 4-H students, siblings, and spouses. And there were Bill and Shirley, married sixty-seven years. Both were soft and round, with bright eyes. Both were in wheelchairs, both holding hands and smiling shyly, both living in the nursing home together.

Jake and his fiancée were going to be okay.

Meeting Jackie and Blurring the Lines

One day, after watching students lead workshops in the Courtyards, I passed the chapel on my way back to my car. The chapel was brimming with music, laughter, and people. By chance, I had stumbled upon the Luther Manor talent show. My first response was shock: Why hadn't the staff, with whom we had monthly check-in calls and who were helping us recruit people to participate in the project, told us that there was a *talent show*?

My second response was awe. I watched as Jean, the activity specialist in the health center, helped a slightly bent older woman with tightly cropped salt-and-pepper hair navigate her way to the stage and take a seat at a keyboard. Jean placed the woman's fingers on the keyboard and went back to her seat. As the woman felt her way around the keyboard to position herself, I realized that she was blind. Suddenly, the keyboard erupted in a buoyant rendition of "Sentimental Journey" and then, on its heels, a flawless "Moon River."

The next day I peppered Jean with questions. Who *was* that? Do you think she would perform in the play? Why didn't you tell me there was a talent show? It turns out that the keyboard player's name was Jackie. And yes, Jean thought that if I asked, Jackie would be happy to play. Jean simply hadn't put it together that the talent show would be of interest. Now she understood. The whole goal of the project was to build on the talents and interests of the community.

Jackie featured prominently in the play, both in the opening and closing scenes. *Finding Penelope*, as you might guess from the title, is the story of the search for Penelope, led by the two main characters, each of a different era. Odysseus, of course, is the stuff of legend and myth. He returns at last to Luther Manor and searches out this strange landscape for his queen. Mira is the "bad" daughter, returned after twenty years of not visiting her mother, Penelope Papadopoulos, who lives in assisted living. Mira is riddled with fear and guilt. Odysseus is puzzled by life in the twenty-first century. Together they help each other navigate the dangers around each bend in the hallway.

The play begins in the lobby area outside Luther Manor's chapel. Looking a bit disheveled, Odysseus enters from the front door like any other guest. When the volunteer ticket-takers check him in, they give him a name tag that reads "Old Beggar." Everyone else, including Mira, gets a name tag that reads "Stranger." After establishing the story line (we are all searching for Penelope), we are guided through heavy double doors and into the hallway of the nursing home by a guitar player and the cast singing "I'm gonna take a sentimental journey . . ." This is a tough entry for the audience. The skilled nursing unit is home to the elders with the most profound disabilities. Their doors are open, and many are in bed, as the forty to fifty performers and audience members stream down the hallway. The jaunty song undercuts the discomfort that you could feel rising among the audience.

Should I look? Do I want to? Am I allowed?

Toward the end of the hallway there is a nurse's station. As the musicians approach it, they quiet their playing. But the song continues. The audience turns the corner to find a small living room area with elders gathered around a television and Jackie, in her pink sweatshirt, seated at her keyboard, picking up where the musicians left off.

Is this part of the performance? Or is this just everyday life in the nursing home?

There was no difference. The audience lingered on the scene, with a heightened interest in the moment: elders in wheelchairs with crocheted lap robes gathered around the television, eyes vaguely taking in an afternoon game show; Jackie, one among them, playing a keyboard, blurring the line between what appeared to be everyday life in the care home and the heightened world of the play itself. Could this simple blurring effect invite audience members to see and experience the care home as a place of possibility and wonder—not just a care home where people pass their time slouched before game shows until they die?

Reading the *Odyssey* in Public

As the project took shape, the Penelope team had monthly conference calls with a good dozen lead collaborators: the director and designer from Sojourn Theatre; the lead staff in each area of care for Luther Manor; and me and my student support team.

"Anyone try any interesting creative workshops over the last month?" I asked in one of our calls. There was a pause, and then Jean, the activity specialist in the skilled nursing area, chimed in. Jean had created a display area for the Penelope project in the nursing home, complete with a mannequin sitting on a chair and weaving on a small loom, a lyre (where on earth did she find a lyre?), and maps of Greece.

"Well, we took a field trip to a nearby lake to see what Penelope might have felt, waiting for her love to return over water," she said.

Wait. You did what?

"It was a beautiful fall day," said Jean. "We read from the *Odyssey*. People were so curious what we were doing."

I can only imagine. A transport van full of older people unloads in a county park. Navigating their walkers, canes, and wheelchairs, they roll up to the lakeside viewpoint, open their copies of the *Odyssey*, and in the warm September light read aloud of Penelope's grieving, for her noble husband and now too her grown son, both at sea, their return uncertain.

What if the project was so interesting that the staff, at all levels, felt empowered to invite the elders to join them in a deep exploration of the themes?

Check.

The Power of High Expectations, or "It's All Greek to Me"

If the gods will grant us
A happier old age
We'll be free from our trials, at last.

These are the last lines of Penelope's story in Homer's *Odyssey*. After the 108 suitors who had taken over the castle are slain and Odysseus passes one final test, the couple is reunited after twenty long years apart. Athena grants them one last gift. She delays the rosy fingers of dawn so that they might linger in each other's company a bit longer.

Classics professor Andrew Porter, a Homeric specialist, joined us one afternoon for a creative workshop in the skilled nursing area. He brought with him a one-page handout with Penelope's last words both in English and in transliterated ancient Greek, which he distributed to the dozen elders gathered in a semicircle in the dining area.

Porter, who was a pastor with an evangelical congregation for years before shifting full-time to the university, used his warm, booming voice to invite the elders to explore the meaning of the passage with him.

"Can you say the words in ancient Greek? Just to see what they feel like in your mouth?"

"Old age. *Gay-ras*," said Porter, with a subtle rolling of the *r*.

Among the elders, there was a chorus of throat-clearing and a few side-eye glances, as if to say, "You want me to do *what*? Speak *ancient Greek*?"

"*Gay-ras.*"

"Great!" Porter is genuinely warmed by their effort and repeats the word with them several times to improve their pronunciation. In a moment captured by the documentary crew that followed the project, Helga turned to the camera and smiled.

"It's all Greek to me," she said grinning.

Dr. Porter visited each of the four areas of care, teaching ancient Greek and exploring key cultural themes in the story, like the command to welcome the stranger, and the concept of *ypoméno*, which translates into English as "endurance," or "remaining under." The staff, artists, and students extended these lively conversations into even more workshops and shared the elders' contributions through photos and notes. Slowly, over the two years, we were all deepening our explorations, building understanding, and transforming our ideas into artistic expression. The list of things the elders said they endured were symbolically slain one by one in the scene in which Odysseus slays the suitors.

What if programming in care settings was incredibly interesting and built over time—even for people with limited time and cognitive disabilities? What if we honored the minds and spirits of staff, elders, and volunteers alike by designing programming that invited learning and expression?

"Can You Create a Weaving Three-Quarters of a Mile Long?"

To mark the route of the play, Sojourn's designer Shannon Scrofano had a special request of the staff. "Can you make a weaving that is as long as the journey we'll take through Luther Manor?" she asked on one of our many conference calls.

There was a long pause. You could see them calculate the distance in their heads. It would be close to three-quarters of a mile. That was *a lot* of weaving. And the first performance was just a month away.

"Yes," said Ellie Rose, a dementia specialist in the day center who also happened to be trained as an artist. "We don't know how, but we'll figure it out."

This was a magical turning point. Until now, the staff tended to want the artists to tell them what to do: "How many people do you want? Where? When? I'll get them there for you." But gradually the openness of our creative process began to become clear. We were all of us making this together. We didn't know what it was going to be any more than the staff did. We had ideas, but so did the staff. The elders, the staff, the artists—we were truly an ensemble, each with our expertise, each crucial to the process.

As it turns out, the staff made the weaving happen. To make the weaving project accessible to a wide range of people, the staff had the idea to use as the base for the weaving the plastic rings around six-packs of cans. After first trying to staple individual rings together, the staff discovered that the rings actually come in long rolls and got a local liquor store to donate a mile's worth. Then the staff cleared out every activity supply closet at Luther Manor for extra fabric and yarn, and they handed out sections of plastic and piles of fabric at every activity session in all four areas of care. People with more dexterity crocheted around the rings. Those with less pulled brightly colored fabric in and out of the plastic circles in a loose weaving.

As time grew short, the staff cut up sections of the rings and made "to-go" kits for staff, students, and volunteers to take home in the evening. Elders could take them back to their rooms as well, to fill any sleepless hours. A week before we opened the first preview, there was a full three-quarters of a mile of weaving in large plastic garbage bags. Activity time was now spent figuring out how to hang the weaving in the hallways without violating the fire code.

The sold-out audiences followed the brightly colored weaving through the hallways, each three-foot panel as unique as every member of the community itself.

Lessons from Luthaca

The play itself was quite a logistical puzzle. We performed at 2 p.m., between lunch and the first rumblings of hunger or habit for dinner. To not overstress the site with crowds, we limited the audience to fifty people. But with the pied-piper effect, the final scene always had nearly seventy-five, drawing residents or staff who followed along with the crowd. The scenes were intense emotionally; this was the *Odyssey* after all. There were always layers of references to life at Luther Manor and life on the ancient island of Ithaca. As the director of the nursing home said in a meeting when I explained the concept, "Ah yes, we are in Luthaca!"

In one scene, a guitar player and singer wove their way through the long hallways of Luther Manor's assisted living area, the Courtyards. Odysseus, still disguised as an Old Beggar to protect him from the 108 suitors, sang a wistful version of Hank Williams's "Rambling Man" to set the pace. They were followed by an audience of fifty people who had paid to see this reimagining of the ancient tale. Odysseus went to war for ten years and took ten years to journey home again. Penelope ruled the kingdom alone for twenty years, raised her son, and fended off the suitors, who took over her castle in an attempt to force her to remarry. Together, the musicians and audience were heading toward a climactic scene in the assisted living dining hall in which Odysseus slays all 108 suitors. They had it coming.

On the way to the dining hall, the performers and audience passed a bulletin board that—like so many bulletin boards in so many care communities—was covered in calendars, seasonal decorations, and inspirational quotes. But on this bulletin board there was also an oddly designed ten-inch square, white sign: "Penelope: Our Cunning, Noble, Wise and Lovely Queen." It was on the next bulletin board too. And the next. Just when the audience started seeing the sign everywhere, someone would say "Penelope," and the audience would find themselves joining in as the actors, the elders, and seemingly everyone standing around them responded in unison: "Our cunning, noble, wise and lovely queen!" Many of the elder residents living along the long corridor had walked or wheeled themselves up to their doorways, watching and waving as the performers and audience members passed by.

Was this part of the show? Who was watching whom?

When the train of audience members arrived at the dining hall, they were welcomed to sit along a long glass wall on one side of the room. On a long bench just behind them sat a dozen elders with memory loss, watching the commotion and doing simple hand gestures in unison.

Was this *part of the show? Who was watching whom?*

This was the scene in *Finding Penelope* in which Odysseus finally sheds his disguise as an old beggar, proving his identity by shooting an arrow through twelve axe-handles. Then, aided by the goddess Athena, he slays the suitors. Odysseus was played by James Hart, a professional actor with Sojourn Theatre. Athena was played by Caroline Imhoff, of the Courtyards. She wore a crown of laurels, rescued from a corner of Luther Manor's basement storage room by the building maintenance director and spray-painted gold by Sojourn's designer, Shannon Scrofano. The suitors were played by just two people, Jake Cohen, a young professional actor in his twenties, and Rusty Tym, a Luther Manor resident who was born for the theater but took seventy-some years to make his professional debut. Both Jake and Rusty wore T-shirts with stencils of fifty-four men on them. Each would menacingly charge Odysseus, only to meet a Three Stooges–style demise. One loses a thumb war. Another gets a lethal poke in the eye or a crushing of the hat. As the suitors are put to rest over and over again, another actor reads from a list of 108 things that Luther Manor residents told us that they endure, much as Penelope endured the suitors and not knowing whether her beloved was dead or alive.

The elders' list contained both the silly and the sublime:

Macular degeneration

Icy sidewalks

Slow elevators

Missing my friends

My annoying sister-in-law

Stroke

Dementia

Guilt

Guilt was the last to go and, with its departure, Mira was free at last to find and visit with her mother—as was the whole audience. With all the suitors dispatched, Odysseus, with his shiny breastplate and bare, muscular arms, led the audience back into the hallways of Luther Manor singing, "Home, let me come home—home is wherever I'm with you." Mira, played by Sojourn's Rebecca Martinez, joined him, buoyant and freed from the weight of being a bad daughter. Both were eager to find Penelope at last—Odysseus his beloved wife, the queen of Ithaca, and Mira her mother. Together they marched the audience joyfully to Luther Manor's chapel, where an array of seats awaited the audience and where an older woman slept peacefully in a golden wheelchair just in front of the chapel's stage, which was hidden by a curtain. Here at last, after Mira and Odysseus had journeyed deep into Luther Manor to find her, was Mira's mother, played by first-time actress Joyce Heinrich. The curtain opened to reveal some thirty elders, some on hospice, some with dementia or stroke or both, all playing Odysseus's queen. Neither Penelope—not the mythic nor the contemporary—recognized their loved one. "Do you know me?" Mira and Odysseus pleaded in unison. Then both of them understood—this isn't really what matters. What matters is that *they* know *her*. Both dig deep, through the layers of fear and sorrow of not being known and the guilt of not being able to fix it, to prove that they know her.

"Penelope, you are my cunning, noble, wise and lovely mother," said Mira.

"Penelope, you are my cunning, noble, wise and lovely queen," said Odysseus.

And with the comfort of feeling truly known, both Penelopes, Mira's mother and the chorus of elders playing Odysseus's queen, extended their arms and welcomed them both home, with movements and words created by the elders themselves:

> My heart is open to you.
> My soul and my spirit welcome you home.
> I am calling you.
> I am hearing you.
> I am seeing you.
> Your eyes sparkle, like the stars.

A New Species of Bird

Director Maureen Towey and I had originally planned for a postshow discussion, but in the preview performances the final scene was met with so much sobbing that we decided on something simpler. Luther Manor staff simply invited the audience up to the stage to share in cookies and conversation with the chorus. The emotions continued on through the cast party after the final performance. With students, artists, elders, staff, and volunteers gathered around, Joyce, who had so beautifully embodied Penelope, shared a fable she'd written to capture the transformative experience.

It all happened one fall afternoon.

The young eagles flew right into the middle of the old crows' nest.

The old crows huddled off to the side and cackled and cawed.

The young eagles puffed their feathers and flapped their wings.

"We've brought you some new food. It's called Penelope."

A few of the old crows ventured forth and nibbled at the edges of the Penelope food. The young eagles stood around and took pictures of the crows and listened to their stories. Soon more crows joined in and then a strange thing happened.

The old crows began to look more like the young eagles as they became more creative, livelier, and enthusiastic. A strange thing also happened to the young eagles as they listened to the wisdom and life stories the old crows offered.

Soon the nest became much bigger.

A new species of bird evolved.

Now they chattered in one voice and the story of the wonderful Penelope food spread throughout the land.

"Did You Enjoy It?"

Truly bringing the staff, elders, and volunteers fully into the creative process turned out to be a seismic shift for the care community. Key stakeholders all gathered for a final focus group meeting two weeks after the final performance, after we'd had a chance to digest all that had happened. Several staff talked about the power of letting go.

"The minute I gave up on trying to control everything was when I started to really enjoy it," said one. Another staff member elaborated:

I think that's a really good thing that we all learned to let go of the control. 'Cause in the beginning we were like, "Where's the schedule? Who is going to do it?" And then . . . the last three weeks we were like, "Just let me know when I'm supposed to show up!" *(laughter in the group)*. And what was really remarkable was to stand back and watch, that as we let go of the control, the residents participated better.

And yet another staff member added: "Yes! To just let it evolve, as it needed to evolve. And to stop trying to superimpose what we thought it should be or what we wanted it to be and rather let it be in the hands of those that were doing it. I think that the delight of the moment was something that I learned."

My UWM colleague and co-instructor Robin, who also played the Nurse in *Finding Penelope*, led the project's evaluation. She went back to Luther Manor a month after the final performance to interview elders who participated. Certainly those in independent living would have vivid memories. But would those in assisted living or skilled care who struggled with memory loss? As she settled in to interview one woman in the skilled care area, Robin wasn't sure what to expect or how exactly to phrase the question. Robin explained that just last month, we had all worked together on the Penelope project. "Did you enjoy it?"

"Oh, yes," she said. "You know, it is the last important thing I will do in my life."

What if care centers really truly became cultural centers? Where activities could build over time to create beauty, meaning, and legacy?

Check.

CHAPTER 11

From Islands to Archipelagos

The awe of the Penelope project lingered in my heart and mind for months. I remember sitting in a Thai restaurant in Brooklyn with Maureen Towey, the director of *Finding Penelope*, months later, still struggling to articulate the emotional power the project had had for us as artists, as people with aging family members, and as people who were, of course, aging ourselves. We also yearned to build on that power. The experience of creating such beauty, with people we weren't sure would live from one performance to the next, had both bonded us and fueled our curiosity. The project worked at Luther Manor, a long-term-care community. Could such a project work with the 95 percent of older people who live at home?

Around the table at that Thai restaurant, Maureen and I began to sketch out the ideas for a project we came to call the Islands of Milwaukee. The goal was to bring meaningful, creative engagement to elders who were living alone at home or who were "underconnected" to their communities. We learned early on in the project that "socially isolated" or "homebound" were not phrases that people wanted to claim for themselves. To reach the underconnected, Maureen and I drew together a network of partners that included Meals on Wheels, a telephone reassurance program, a volunteer friendly-visit program, and a home-care agency.

After months of partnership building, Maureen and I found ourselves and two other artists from Sojourn Theatre one autumn morning at the Beulah Brinton Community Center, nestled in the heart of Bayview, on Milwaukee's south side. The center was just ten blocks from where my father grew up, in a classic, two-bedroom Milwaukee bungalow that my great-grandfather had built. My dad's mother had grown up there, raised my father there, and aged there until Grandpa's smoking and lung disease caught up with him and they had to move to an apartment near us. But Grandma's roots in Bayview were too deep. Replanted, she never took hold, and both of them were gone in just two years. The Beulah Brinton Community Center is in the heart of my grandmother's deeply lived neighborhood. Young mothers gather with their toddlers for playtime. People of all ages make the old wooden floors squeak as they play competitive volleyball. Elders from the neighborhood gather around long tables for conversation over lunch.

The Beulah Brinton Community Center is also a dispatch site for Meals on Wheels, delivering hundreds of meals each day to elders in the neighborhood who can't make it to the center. The drivers gathered there were all business, checking charts, and packing meals. Our team of four artists were there for a "ride-along," to observe what the drivers do firsthand to see whether we could insert creative engagement into their daily interactions. We had just come from making magic happen with the Penelope project. We knew we could bring meaning and connection to a care community, where staffing and daily routines provided infrastructure for creativity. But bringing meaning and connection to people in their homes would be a bigger lift. We'd need to figure out how to deliver the spark and how to gather it back. To connect each person to a larger purpose, we would have to figure out how to build on the person's responses and then once again share our response back. And every single person we tried to engage could easily say no. A stranger at my door or on my phone? Asking me to be creative? I would probably say no if it were me.

But the urgency for us to try to create this distribution system for meaningful engagement was profound. More older people than ever are living alone. And social isolation, research tells us, is the health risk equivalent of fifteen cigarettes a day.[1] So many people claim to want to stay in their own homes as they age. But when that means living alone, the physical and psychological costs can be tremendous, both for individuals and for communities. Consider the 1995 heat wave in Chicago: 739 people died of heat-related causes—most of them older adults, living alone. In Milwaukee that same summer, 154 people died of heat-related causes. The telephone reassurance system we were partnering with on this project was created in part to ensure this never happened again.

As lead artists, Maureen and I introduced our team to the drivers, who were polite but barely looked up as they rhythmically sorted and checked and packed. We tried to be helpful.

"Can I carry anything?"

"No, I got it."

We quickly learned that what was really helpful was stepping back and letting the drivers get into the flow of loading a hundred meals into their cars. I was to ride along with Mr. John Robertson, who went by Johnny. He had a warm smile and serious demeanor. As he was my senior by thirty-some years, I opted to call him Mr. Johnny. I asked whether I should ride with him in his truck or follow behind in my car. "You can follow behind me," he said matter-of-factly.

In Milwaukee, Meals on Wheels drivers are paid, not volunteers, although the pay is really just enough to offset the cost of gas. The drivers clearly do this work because they want to help people, and Mr. Johnny clearly loved helping the people on his route. He had the same determined flow when he drove as he did loading the meals; I had to be on my toes. He would cross multiple lanes of traffic to make a turn that would shorten the route by thirty seconds. I thought I knew the neighborhood. But he knew every alley, every shortcut. We stopped at houses and apartment buildings, some neat and trim, some not. At each one, I would hop out and follow him up to the door—sometimes the front, sometimes the back. He would ring the doorbell or knock; he knew what was most effective for each person. The door would open surprisingly quickly. I understood better why the drivers were rushing to start their deliveries: they were expected.

Almost every engagement was the same. There was a warm greeting, about thirty or forty seconds of banter about the weather or sports, a heartfelt inquiry with a genuine expectation of response: "How are you doing?" Somehow Mr. Johnny never seemed rushed during this exchange. He would hand the person a foil-topped black box with the meal inside; on this day it was a medley of wax and green beans, potato casserole, a roll, a pat of butter, something called

Salisbury steak, a cookie, and orange juice. Mr. Johnny also handed the person a little blue envelope that the person could return with a donation inside the next time Mr. Johnny visited.

"Do people really give donations?" I asked.

"Sometimes," he told me. "They'll save up and once a month I might get a few dollars. It means a lot to them to be able to give me something in return."

At some apartment buildings, he pulled out a little wheeled cart and loaded multiple meals into it. I was struck that we sometimes delivered meals at apartments next door to each other. At each, the door would open, Mr. Johnny and the person would have a friendly exchange, and the door would close. You had the sense that the door never opened again until the next time he knocked. And yet, these two people were just next door to each other.

Mr. Johnny would share some of his concerns and highlights with me as we walked down the hallways. "This gentleman down here's wife just passed. I'm worried about him." Or "Oh, you're going to love Tony, he was a schoolteacher."

At one stop, we pulled into a parking lot between two abandoned stores. Around the side of one of the buildings I could see a trailer park hidden from the main street.

"Don't come with me to this one," he said, quietly and firmly.

I stayed in the car.

At another stop, a woman in her forties answered the door. Mr. Johnny asked whether her mother was home. "Yeah, I'll give it to her." He reluctantly handed her the tray.

"Sometimes they never get the meal," he said as we walked back to our cars.

We pulled up to another house and knocked. No response. Mr. Johnny looked nervous. He peeked in the window. He told me to wait while he went around the back. He reemerged, on his cell phone. If someone doesn't answer the door as expected, the drivers notify the main office, and someone will call or come out later to check on the person. He paused once more at the door, and then we were back into the flow. We still had a good dozen meals to deliver.

This same scene plays itself out with four or five drivers at nine different dispatch sites all across Milwaukee County: two thousand meals a day. Fridays are extra busy, as multiple frozen meals are delivered to get people through the weekend.

The artists gathered over lunch and talked about the possibilities. We had around forty drivers delivering some two thousand meals a day. In many cases, the driver was the only person the elder saw each day. We had thirty to forty seconds at the door—less in the dead of winter when no one wants to open the door for long. We had a blue envelope that was dropped off and later picked up and returned to the main office. We had dispatch site directors who were the liaisons to the main office.

We needed something fast and simple that didn't burden the drivers. No one had computers or tablets, or Wi-Fi for that matter. And if we gave people tablets, we'd be making already vulnerable elders into targets for robbery. But almost everyone had phones, and we learned that the county had a program that subsidized cell phones for people who didn't have them.

How would we introduce ourselves? We couldn't ask the meal recipients to make "art" with us. Art was too hard to explain, and people had too many misconceptions of it. We needed a simple invitation that was low risk and intriguing. We decided we would simply give the drivers a question to ask: "I have a Question of the Day. Would you like to hear it?" We designed and printed forty-five Question of the Day cards, which were the size of index cards and could fit right on top of the meal. They were poetic, playful, and thoughtful. They invited people to think about their day, their home, their neighborhood, themselves, a little differently—and from a position of strength.

The next puzzle was to figure out how we could gather responses. Based on the information we gathered in our ride-alongs, we created a voice-mail line for people to call in their responses. We also created a question box at each dispatch site where drivers could drop any handwritten responses they gathered, not unlike that blue envelope.

In eight months, we received more than two thousand responses from just two pilot dispatch sites.

The project was slow to start, with drivers unsure whether this was worth their while. But when we stopped back at the Beulah Brinton Community Center six months later, the drivers regaled us with stories of their favorite responses. They loved reading the handwritten cards. Some were written in careful cursive. Some looked breezy. With others, you could imagine the person pushing through arthritis pain to make the looping letters.

What could you teach another person?

"To care for the elderly, to be kind, to give your troubles to Jesus."

"To organize things."

If you could go anywhere right now, where would you go?

"To see the house I grew up in."

"The Red Lobster. I have a craving for crab."

"To the YMCA to take a shower."

"To the art museum."

What's the most beautiful sound in your home?

"The dishwasher. It has always calmed me, even as a child."

What is your safe harbor?

"My easy chair, with a glass of scotch."

Angie left voice-mail responses to every single question. Chelsea, one of the graduate students working with us on the project, called her back to thank her for her responses and asked whether she might want to receive what we called an "artistic house call," a follow-up visit to go a little deeper into creativity. Angie lived in a subsidized senior apartment complex on the south side of Milwaukee. She was intrigued by the prospect of an artistic house call, and when Chelsea asked what kind of art she might want to make, Angie said, "Finger painting." So, a week later, Chelsea made her way to the south side with painting supplies and later emerged with several paintings. Several years later, one of those paintings would win Angie an award through a regional disability arts contest.

With more than two thousand written and recorded responses, we were clearly succeeding at gathering responses. But meaningfulness is predicated on having a connection to the world beyond you, so we wanted to ensure that the people who shared their answers to the Questions of the Day with us knew that we were building on their answers and that they were being honored and heard. We wanted to offer proof of listening. Chelsea, who had some serious design skills, digitally captured the handwriting on each card and created posters of all the responses that we sent back out with the drivers. We worked with a sound artist and editor to create twenty-one radio segments inspired by interviews and voice-mail messages. We formed a partnership with WUWM, Milwaukee's public radio station, and aired weekly segments for the project, hoping that the meal recipients would hear their voices.

Finally, as the culminating event for the project, we created an art installation at City Hall, featuring listening stations where visitors could hear soundscapes remixed from the radio segments and see the handwritten cards at "question stations," where visitors could also add their own response card to the display. We opened the exhibit with a performance in which local actors, blended with those from our partner Sojourn Theatre, read aloud some of the more poignant responses from various levels of the historic City Hall atrium. The performance ended with one of the actors asking, "I have a Question of the Day— would you like to hear it?" That was my cue. I had a cardboard box filled with hundreds of Question of the Day cards. I inched my way over to the edge of the railing—eight floors is quite vertigo-inducing—and gently shook the box to release the cards. They looked like a light Milwaukee snow, slowly fluttering down from the top floor and into the waiting hands of the audience.

What is courage to you?

How are you courageous in your daily life?

What does it mean to be a hero?

Who is a hero to you?

What is something you would like to learn?

Where do you connect to nature?

Thousands of Question of the Day cards now reside in my basement. I dream of working with a designer to create an exhibit that can travel to libraries and meal sites across the country so others can experience the personality in the careful curving cursive letters and add their own voices to the dialogue started with hundreds of elder Milwaukeeans. The TimeSlips team has begun conversations with the national Meals on Wheels program to bring our model and its lessons learned to a handful of the independently run Meals on Wheels programs across the country.

I have a Question of the Day. Would you like to hear it?

What if one day, every meal is delivered with a little added nutrition for the soul—an invitation to shape the world with a bit of poetry or a story?

CHAPTER 12

Bill Teaches Me About Time (and Rocks)

Bill lived in a fortress of freshly constructed senior living apartments where the lobbies have soaring ceilings and bright banks of windows that overlook carefully tended grounds. These are the buildings lauded in glossy marketing pamphlets for care settings in the United States. When you walk through them, though, these buildings can feel a bit like libraries without books, with residents sitting wordless, watching the groundskeepers, the banter of staff discussing something—construction on the nearby access road—muffled behind the reception desk. A joke and laughter are quickly self-hushed.

Up at Bill's second-floor apartment, a home-care attendant welcomed me at the door, the sound of the television bouncing off the walls. She was happy to see me, but our warm greetings overlap and interrupt each other as I tried to encourage her to stay and she explained something about needing to run an errand and being right back. I was alone as I stepped through the small entryway and into the living room. Bill was sleeping in a recliner a bit too close to the wall. A line of brown smudges and gashes in the drywall behind him seemed to mark his days in the chair. It was my third visit, so he wouldn't be startled to find me there when he woke. I waited.

I had been coming to see Bill every few weeks for an "artistic house call" as part of the Islands of Milwaukee project. One of our partners on the project was a home-care agency interested in learning how creative engagement might be integrated into the agency's training and care systems. I offer the story of my experiences with Bill, in the hope that it might do just that: provide a window into what the growing home-care industry might look like if the scaffolding of meaning and shared creativity were built into it.

In my first visit with Bill, my goal was simply introductions. I wanted to get a feel for who he had been and who he was now—gathering cues from the objects in the room, his caregiver, and conversations with Bill himself. The tiny living room was sparse but stately, dark wood furniture holding thick coffee-table books about boats, ships, and waterways. Nautical artifacts weighed down the room—heavy brass objects whose functions I could only guess. I feel waves of nausea just saying the word "boat."

In that first week, the care manager had introduced me. "I'm here to invite you to imagination," I said, checking to see whether that explanation resonated in some way. "Just to talk a while and share stories." His eyes brightened, he seemed game. But slowly, and with great determination and concentration, he cautioned me.

"I can't (*10 seconds*) speak (*stuttering and more seconds*) very (*again*) well (*tremendous sense of accomplishment*)."

Suddenly I recognize one of those heavy brass objects holding down the coffee table. It's a clock.

The brightness behind Bill's eyes has a nearly impossible journey to make to manifest itself, across the tremendous temporal dissonance between his world and the world of the clock, the world of "time's up!" game-show buzzers and the gossip of daytime talk shows—the world outside the walls of this fortress, where the steady hum of cars flouting the speed limit on the interstate is like an impenetrable moat. Bill is slow. The world is fast.

Temporal dissonance. Recognizing it and calibrating it are crucial to connecting fully with another person but, with the imperialism of institutional time, often nearly impossible. Things simply have to get done. Shifts need to change. Pills need to be distributed. Home is where we control our own sense of time. Feeling unable to step into rapid conversations or briskly moving bodies and carts can lead people to withdraw into the comfort of their own temporal reality and, in turn, isolation.

So I tossed out my agenda, and I slowed down.

"I have a Question of the Day," I say. "Would you like to hear it?"

"Of course," he said, smiling. I smiled too—although I wasn't sure whether this would work, whether his struggle to get words into the world would frustrate him into silence.

The Questions of the Day emerged out of the Islands of Milwaukee project, which I co-led with Maureen Towey of Sojourn Theatre. In the weeks that I visited Bill, the Question of the Day was smack dab in the middle of a three-part series. "What is a well-worn path in your home?" was followed by "What is a well-worn path outside your home?" and then "What blocks your path?"

"What is a well-worn path outside your home?" I asked and showed him the card so he could read it as well.

Bill closed his eyes, and a slow grin grew across his face. What had I stumbled into?

It's difficult to convey our conversation in written form. On my recordings, you can hear the tremor of his hands and steady labor of his breath. There are thick pauses and stutters, some staccato with forward motion, some gummy, stopping up the flow of sound and thought. Sometimes after a long pause, he would sigh, his shoulders sinking in resignation. He is working so hard. If our discussion together had been animated, you would see the gears and wheels turning and smoking with his thoughts. But in the unanimated version, it was just Bill, eyes closed, hands shaking, willing his breath to turn to words, summoning every ounce of strength toward relaying a story of something he clearly and deeply loved. I describe the reality here so you can apply it to the passages that follow, which reveal the treasure of another human being, emerging in glorious fullness, in his own time.

> As you climb up this path, when you get to the top of the path and you look back down you've got a lake—a view of the lake. The lake, lake, lake Michigan. When you get to the top there is a road. And it's going away from the path that goes up the hill. And as you walk along this path, the path leads away from the hillside top. (*Breath. Frustration. Quiet.*)

"It's okay," I told him, "just take us with you wherever you are going."

Well, for years I would follow this path and eventually I would get out to the road, going backwards from there. The path, the path heads through this field. And this picture shows *(pointing to a series of photos on his wall)*—it's kind of hard to understand. The first picture describes this path. But. The. Ah.

"So this is up by your summer home?"

Yeah. And as you walk along this path, it's it's it's . . . It starts from the top of the path through this field and the . . . and the . . . and the path itself. *(Pause.)* Leads away from the edge of this path. *(Long silence.)*

"How does the path make you feel?"

Special. And it makes me feel curious too. Because the path itself—*(pause)*—follows through this field.

"And you are curious where it goes?"

Yes—be-be-because for years, for seventy years roughly, I followed this path which three three three years ago there was a—*(pause; sound of shaking)*—

"Where was your summer home, can I ask?"

Charlevoix, Michigan.

"Charlevoix? Overlooking the lake?"

Oh yeah. The the the path—I'm not doing a good job of describing it.

"It's okay," I said.

> The size of the path was not any longer once you got on this path at the top of the hill. You got to the top of this hill. Every year, I'd walk by all I could see of the path about ten feet wide. And *(pause)*—I always wondered where it led to. Grass had grown on both sides of the path. *(Pause.)* All I could see was about. *(Long pause.)* Oh man.

Again I told him, "It's okay." I was trying to show that I was listening with my face, my words, my posture—my whole self.

> I decided one summer, it was about three summers ago, that I wanted to see how wide it really was. So I got a shovel and a hoe and I started digging. And my brother would walk by about every hour and see how I was doing. And some of our kids that were up there were stopping and asking how's the project doing *(chuckles)* and by the end of the second day, the uh, *(pause)*—
>
> So so we had started digging and then one by one some friends joined us. And some people would say, would laugh and say, you are probably never going to find how deep it is. So so the ah. *(Pause.)* So the start of the path—*(pause)*—the path—*(pause)*.

"Was it surprising?"

> Very. When we finally stopped digging, we had to dig all around it. And then start pulling away from from from the main hole. We could see we were never going—*(pause)*—we can shortcut this by-ssss. And so we got our tractor out and chains and before you know we had enough chain to get around the rock. And the rock was I'll call it the beginning of the hole. And one of our neighbors. Um.

(Pause. Long pause.)

I'm beginning to think I picked a devil of a subject . . .

I laughed. "I work in the land of metaphor," I said, "so I am fasci-nated."

Well, this this this now leads to—why just that hole?
Why don't I start exposing more rocks?

"So when do you stop?"

Well, that's what my children were asking.

So this is a project every summer. I'm the only one
doing it because everyone else thinks I'm a nut. That's.
Most of the holes, they um. *(Pause.)* One of the rocks
we unearthed turned out to be about the shape of the
state of Michigan.

"But smaller?" I smiled. He smiled.

Yeah. Smaller version of Michigan. So the rocks that we
pull out of the vvvv-various holes, some were attractive
enough that I was allowed to place it in spots. So if you
were in Charlevoix, you'd find them maybe ten or fifteen
or twenty scattered throughout the premises.

"The physical labor of doing that had to be enormous."

Well, yes, but it's not as bad as you think because you can
sssss-see. It's. The soil up there is very sandy. So it made
made the digging fairly easy. And I got this great sense
of satisfaction because I had exposed this rock—well—
there's *(pause)*—there's at least twenty-five or thirty more

rocks that I could attack and raise out of the ground. My kids got concerned about their inheritance *(laughter)*— well, at one point I called a local contractor who had a, had a fancy hole fork—and he could stick it into the ground and in about one hour get a hole like that. And he'd say, "Bill, tell me where you'd like this rock to go." For instance, that rock was probably the size of a Volkswagen. He he he. *(Long pause. Breathing.)*

"How did those rocks make you feel?"

I had, ah. *(Pause.)* I, I felt like I had exposed a part of the history of the farm. Um. *(Pause.)* I brought this rock back to life. *(Pause.)* My wife thought I was nuts. The place today, this this this created some character to the place. These these rocks turn the clock back maybe two hundred years. The farmer whoever it was at the time had spent an awful lot of time and sweat *(pause)*, digging rocks in the woods, tracking the, tracking them— and *(pause)* ssss ssss—the farmer, the farmers, there were two farmers—*(pause)*—those farmers did what I did but for different reasons. One just to clear their fields so they can grow more crops. Me, I had done it for an aesthetic reason I guess. So we could look at them alongside the roadside.

"What do you think it is you like so much about rocks?"

I, I, I, I think it's because *(laughing)* rocks accept me as I am *(laughing)*.

Rocks don't talk back to me.

Rocks were all—there's no such thing as a new rock. All the rocks I know of have been on this earth God knows how long. Huh.

(Pause. Long pause.)

"Writers, they use words so generations from now can know what they thought," I told him. "But you were using rocks, which are much heavier than words . . . (*laughter*)." I told him that future generations would be able to read what he wrote on the landscape.

> Yes. *(Pause.)* If we move forward, another hundred years, well in a way I forgot the obvious, the farmer then might decide to fill the hole back up. Which I guess makes me kind of sad.

"Thank you for working so hard to tell that story," I told him. "It's a fascinating story."

> Well, you are the first one that asked me the hard questions.

I think back to the moment of walking into the apartment. A story of two hundred years of farmers moving rocks. The cycle of history and time and our place in it and the crazy reasons we do things. All unearthed by a single beautiful question, listening, and waiting. I certainly had not expected that today.

But I could also feel the pressure of that brass clock. I could feel the menace of temporal imperialism. I looked at my phone. I didn't want to, but I had to. My time was up. I needed to drive the thirty minutes back to campus, find parking, teach class. The students would be waiting for me.

Bill Rings Through

When I returned a few weeks later, I practically ran through the hushed lobby, around the corner through the dining area and up the elevator to the second floor, slowing down only when I entered Bill's time zone. I was eager to hear more about the farm, but I tried to match his pace. Our Question of the Day this week is perfect for him: "What are the sounds of your neighborhood?" He and I laughed our way through chicken "boks," horse "clops," and pig "slurps." Perhaps because words were so hard, he relished the sounds, unafraid to be silly and play with me. But it was when he started to describe the rituals on the farm after meals that the real magic unfolded. It wasn't easy. I asked about the sounds of cutting the grass and hay, and his gears gummed up as he tried to answer.

> Well, they did that. They planted the. They planted the seed in the fall and around June 20th or 30th they would *(pause)*. They would hook the *(pause)*—the *(pause; eyes shut with concentration)*—the whirring sound of the cutter followed by the whirring sound of the cutter cutting them. *(Long pause.)* Oh boy.

"It's hard," I said.

> (Pause.) *Let's keep going.*

"What about the sounds?" I asked. "Do you have a sound in mind, or can I ask you a question? I don't want to interrupt your train of thought."

> I have songs of the farm. In the evening, after dinner, we'd we'd all gather in the great room and Grandfather would bring his guitar and he'd sing—
>
> *(singing)* "Oh, the Lord took a rib from Adam's side, he made a woman and the woman she died. Pharaoh's army got drowned, oh Mary don't weep."

I was truly floored. Bill's voice was a strong, soothing, melodious tenor that floated out of him without hesitation, without any hint of tremor. I was relieved my shock doesn't register and that he continued.

> Song after song and my brother would come in later and he would play. I don't know where our album is. We did a ten-inch long-play record that only a mother would like.

"Did you play guitar too?"

> No, I just sang. Steve played guitar and composed five or six songs. And then the rest would be *(singing)* "Swing low, sweet chariot."

I told him that I could sing that one with him if he wanted. I had grown up singing that at camp.

Together we cleared our throats and laughed. We had to warm up a bit.

> "Swing low . . ."

When we finished the chorus, Bill looked around the empty room mischievously, and asked "Anybody out there want to sing a verse?"

We sang the song again. The strength and smoothness of his voice were remarkable. As fun as the singing was, he turned the conversation back to the sounds of the farm. He told me that the most emotional sound was no sound at all. Their farm was seasonal. And at the end of the summer, as the last car, filled with kids and grandkids, was heading out of the driveway, he and his brother Steve would just stand there, watching the dust rise. He could hear the sound of kids crying in the yard first, wanting to stay longer. The dog would race down the driveway after the cars when she realized what was happening—that she'd have to wait until next spring to play with them again.

> And then we just stood there. If it was a windy day, then you had leaves blowing. But if you had a nice calm day, the cars would head up the hill to this second tier of roads and out toward the bigger road. And they disappeared over the bluff, and we saw some dust and ah—then we'd just stand there and wait. And we'd look and get a little teary-eyed because now there was no sound at all. And it was distinct— I don't know, I can't think of the word. But they *(pause)*— but no sound is sometimes—it's kind of lonely. *(Pause.)* There were some distinct sounds, but then all of a sudden, nothing.

Sometimes, Gears Fail

On the next visit, the gears were even gummier. The Question of the Day, "What are the sounds of your city?" sent him deep inside his mind, so deep it was nearly impossible for the words to surface. I tried to prompt him a bit, asking if there were sounds near where he kept his boat. He was silent for a long time, and then said:

> In my mind I'm driving around the city and *(pause)* trying to connect. *(Another long pause.)*

"Are you still driving?" I asked. I'm trying so hard to prompt him—sounds of water on the boat? He was quiet. Deep in thought, it was hard to pull the thoughts together and the words from the thoughts.

> **Boat sounds, the sound of water slapping on the hull.**
> *(Pause. Long pause. Opens eyes.)* **I'm afraid I'm not a very good customer.**

"I'm just enjoying living in the moment when you are going to these places," I said, "and how hard you are trying." It was just too torturous, so I retold some of the stories from last week and thanked him for trying so hard.

"That Is Really Good"

When I returned again, I resolved to go to the place of his greatest ease and strength: music. I brought my guitar, and the lyrics and chords to "Rock of Ages," but pretty quickly we abandoned both, singing a cappella and coming up with our own lyrics. We gathered words and themes from our conversations: Rocks. Silence. Generations. Petoskey stones. We filled in colors and feelings. Doreen, the care manager from the home-care company, was sitting in the kitchen, listening, filling pill bottles, trying not to disturb us as we went deep into creative flow, trying out and casting aside multiple versions of lyrics.

"Gray Petoskey stones?" I said.

"Shades of gray Petoskey stones?" he countered.

There was a glimmer in his eyes when he told me his theory—that so many tourists collected the stones that, in five hundred years, geologists will be very confused to find all the Petoskey stones in rock gardens in Detroit and Chicago.

We sang, rewrote, sang again.

"Once more from the top," he said.

Sang, rewrote, and sang again, until we landed on this:

Rock of Ages, cleft for me
Let me hide myself in thee
As generations ebb and flow
Your silence it unfolds
Shades of gray Petoskey stones
On the shores of Charlevoix

Doreen chimed in from the kitchen, "That is really good."

I was thinking the same thing.

"Can I just say thank you?" I said. "Because this was really fun." His laugh was warm and full, like his tenor. As we went to record it one last time, I told him that the pitch was a little high for me, but I can fake it.

"Well," he said, with his mischievous glimmer, "as you get toward the end (*pause*) . . . you can just scream."

I made several recordings of Bill singing his songs of the farm and invited a professional sound designer to layer it with voices of volunteers from the project, adding harmony. We featured it in an installation with all the stories from the Islands of Milwaukee in City Hall, where thousands of people got to experience Bill's melodious voice. I brought the recordings back to him one last time so he could enjoy them too.

And I brought him a rock: not a Petoskey stone but a keepsake rock that my youngest son had gathered on one of our walks to Lake Michigan. How could I not?

What if home-care workers, Meals on Wheels drivers, and home-visit volunteers, who are so often alone with an elder, felt like part of a larger, meaningful project?

What if together they could build bridges across isolation—bridges made of imagination and expression?

CHAPTER 13

Let Voices Ring

Light was pouring into the sanctuary of the First Congregational Church in Appleton, Wisconsin, on an April afternoon in 2016. The parking lot was full, and when my sons and I look for a spot to sit, we have to go all the way to the front. We settle in to the third row, just behind two rows of people wearing sky-blue T-shirts that say, "On a Positive Note." This is just one of the three choirs that are gathering here today. The dozen or so members of On a Positive Note are drawn from visitors to one of the nine "memory cafes" in the area, known as the Fox Valley. This event, the choirs, and the cafes are all part of the Fox Valley Memory Project, founded by John and Susan McFadden with the dream of making a supportive community for people living with dementia.

Just over two hundred thousand people live in the midsize towns that dot the banks of the Fox River as it widens into lakes and narrows to cut through limestone. These waters fueled the once booming timber and paper industries here in towns like Appleton, Neenah, Menasha, Oshkosh, and, furthest south, Fond du Lac, with names that echo their Native and French pasts.

Appleton is the cultural center of the valley, with Lawrence University and its nationally recognized music conservatory fueling generations of interest in the arts of all kinds. Having grown up just thirty minutes away, my mom went to Lawrence. It is a cluster of stately, cream-colored brick buildings along the bluff above the Fox River, in the heart of the still-thriving downtown. She begged me to go there, but I had drawn a circle around the Midwest and picked colleges (just like Lawrence) outside of that circle. I wanted out. Now I'm back.

My husband was out of town, and so I flat-out bribed my boys, then fourteen and eleven, to make the two-hour drive with me so I wouldn't miss this event. At the time, I knew of only one other chorus for people with dementia, The Unforgettables, and it was in New York City.[1] This was little Appleton, Wisconsin, where John and Susan's passion for building a place where families with dementia could feel the supportive net of their community had brought together three choruses into one building.

It was a Sunday, the only day my emergent teenagers had to sleep in, so my bribe had to be pretty inspired. The older one, Ben, had a budding interest in photography and had received a fancy camera for Hanukkah earlier that year. "I will pay you to photograph the event," I told him. The kid loves money. "And you guys can watch movies in the car." Not a single grimace or harrumph. We were off.

My husband is a documentary filmmaker, and so the boys are used to seeing their dad capture events. Their response is a mixture of

horror at how close he will get to the main action (once, when film-
ing a friend's outdoor wedding, he crouch-walked up the aisle, laid
down on his belly at the couple's feet, and panned upward), on the one
hand, and comfort with melting in and capturing the moment, on
the other.

Ben took a few shots from our seats in the third row but then got
up and moved around to the side for a better view. On a Positive Note
was first up. They began with "Goodnight, My Love."

Goodnight, my love
Pleasant dreams and sleep tight, my love
May tomorrow be sunny and bright
And bring you closer to me

The words thickened with meaning as caregivers and spouses
watched loved ones in the sky-blue T-shirts singing to the packed
church.

If you should awake in the still of the night
Please have no fear
For I'll be there, darling, you know I care
Please give your love to me, dear, only

This was quite a choice. Ben snuck in behind the piano, following
the lead of the photographer from the local paper, and focused his
lens on the group. The choir followed up with "Sweet Betsy from
Pike," "Oh! Susanna," and "Show Me the Way to Go Home"—more
crowd-pleasing sing-along than emotional double entendre, although

"Show Me the Way to Go Home," sung by people with memory loss, might also have represented some good old-fashioned dark humor.

Next up were the Memory Care Singers. Residents and family members from five area nursing homes had been practicing songs for weeks. Now they were all seated together, with staff interspersed, in a whole section of the pews. "April Showers," "Look for the Silver Lining," "By the Light of the Silvery Moon"—these were sing-along classics, and the whole room filled with song. We were less listening to a choir and more joining in a group sing led by residents of local nursing homes. "You Are My Sunshine"—everyone in the room swayed and clapped. My younger son and I put our arms around each other and joined our row in swaying. I used to sing this song in the car to calm the kids when they were little. I still sing this song. Then it was "And the Band Played On," followed by a roof-raising version of "Amen."

Ben struggled with overcoming some polite shyness, but he found some lovely moments. What drew him to a shot? What was he seeing? Feeling?

Last up was the big show, the NewVoices Choir. They rose from their seats and spread out across the front of the church, an impressive bunch, thirty or forty people deep. These were the pros, directed by the head of Choral Studies at Lawrence University, and beloved in the Appleton community since 1978. They could easily blow the roof off the place with fancy interpretations of anything from medieval madrigals to Broadway show tunes. But several years ago, the New-Voices Choir turned to deliberate community engagement—a genuine meeting of music and everyday people's lives and concerns. This year the NewVoices Choir chose to collaborate with the Fox Valley Memory Project. The choir selected "Home on the Range," "Amazing Grace," and "Blue Skies," closing with "Over the Rainbow," inviting the whole room to sing along as the choir added multiple, gorgeous layers of harmony.

There is nothing like the power of a group sing—all voices joining together, shared breathing between lines, harmony rising throughout the room. *Who is that? Who knows the harmony?* You look around but can't tell. We were all one—inhaling and exhaling with sound and rhythm, with words we all knew by heart, without fear of forgetting. It is truly a moment of awe—that together we can create something so beautiful that rises above our worries, our losses, our grief. Awe that John and Susan have built this community event with such patience, attention to detail, and love.

Of course, I cry. I always cry in group sings. I love to sing but I was never able to join a chorus, or step onto the singer-songwriter path I longed for, because of the weeping. My sister, a trained singer, had a recital in college that I attended. She opened her mouth, something loud and Italian came out, and I burst into tears. It was something about the strength and beauty of the voice just pouring out of her. Something perhaps about breathing and singing being so close to praying. Perhaps tears are just my reaction to awe.

My younger son, Will, looked up and smiled at me: *Yep, she's crying.* He knew I would be. He snuggled into my shoulder a little more.

When we got home, Ben uploaded his pictures to the computer. He caught some lovely moments. In the photos I can see his caution to get too close: Is it respect? Or fear? But I can also see the awe. Around the corners of people's eyes and mouths, you can read the calm joy of knowing what to say, of knowing they can participate fully. I think of the last line of "Over the Rainbow," the very last song of the concert: "Why, oh why can't I?"

But here, they can. We all can.

"Not a Sing-Along"

Mary Lenard, executive director of Giving Voice Chorus in Minneapolis, is adamant that the chorus is *not* a sing-along group. "Sing-alongs are great," she tells me, "but these choirs involve learning new music and performing in large-scale public venues"—like St. Paul's ornate Ordway Theater, where the chorus performed *Love Never Forgets* in June 2018, featuring original music inspired by members' own stories and shaped into songs by lyricist Louisa Castner and composer Victor Zupanc.[2] Mary and her cofounder, Marge Ostrouschko, began the Giving Voice Chorus in 2014 out of a desire to honor their parents who had struggled with dementia. Mary had been the executive director of the Alzheimer's Association Minnesota–North Dakota Chapter, and so she was well aware of the challenges faced by people who were striving to live at home rather than move to a care setting—like isolation, depression, and paralyzing stigma. They also knew of Jeanie Brindley-Barnett's work as cofounder of the MacPhail Music for Life program at MacPhail Center for Music in Minneapolis. Jeanie was working magic with the Sing for Life chorus of older men and women. Mary and Marge decided that their tribute to their parents would be a chorus for people with dementia, and brought in Jeanie as music director for a pilot year.

To kick-start the chorus, Mary worked her connections with the caregiver groups at the Alzheimer's Association chapter. When they gathered for their first of fourteen weeks of rehearsal, there were thirty people in the room: people with dementia, caregivers, and volunteers alike. Helen Kivnick, a renowned gerontologist, was among them. Helen began her career working with Erik and Joan Erikson and had developed her own focus on vital involvement. I had been lucky enough to have Helen on my dissertation committee (so long ago now) and was eager to reconnect and interview her about her experiences with Giving Voice. "At first I sang with the baritones because that's where they needed me," she said. "I had to sing their part in their range—which posed interesting challenges for me." Helen participated, observed, and conducted interviews with a research assistant to evaluate the pilot. When I asked her for her general observations, she said, "Being in a choir activates everything wonderful about music and music making and everything good about being part of a group where everyone has active ownership. Every participant engages in growth and mastery, being helpful and being helped. And the audiences can't believe what they see and hear."

What really struck Helen about Giving Voice, though, was how it made her think about disability. "What I kept being reminded of is how everybody who is alive has both disabilities and abilities. I see that no place more clearly than in this choir," said Helen. That first pilot had people with fairly advanced dementia, including two women with aphasia, which corrupts one's ability to speak. But they could both sing in the choir. One of them told Helen's research assistant that if she had a psychotherapy session after rehearsal, sometimes she could still talk. Her partner said she had fallen in love with this woman because of her voice. Being in the choir enabled her partner to hear that voice every single week and to fall in love with her all over again.

Like Mary, Helen saw the power of Giving Voice in its rigorous expectations. These were two-hour rehearsals over fourteen weeks with a professional music director. Jeanie Brindley-Barnett was adamant that participants would not be infantilized with low expectations. "We are going to treat our people like we treat ourselves," she said. Yet, while she had vast experience working with older adult choirs, she had never worked with a chorus made up primarily of people with dementia. She was in new territory. "How much new material can we present?" she wondered. She decided that the group could handle new music as long as it "resonated with their heart and soul." And that resonance would come through in performances.

Brindley-Barnett decided to aim high but to make the rehearsal process accessible to everyone. Some could read music, some couldn't. So she always made recordings available for people to learn parts by listening, as well as the traditional music. She told me a story that reinforced her impulse. They were halfway through their first fourteen-week session when Ken raised his hand. Jeanie knew that he had played in his high school band, and maybe even college, but he could no longer read music because of his dementia. But in rehearsal, Jeanie said, "Ken raised his hand and, looking at his sheet music, he said, "'Wait a minute—you said F-sharp, but I don't have that.' He was reading music again!"

Even Jeanie was surprised by the group's capacity and hunger to learn. "They want to bring it to a higher level," she said, "and they have. Their sight reading is a miracle to me. We are doing three- and four-part harmony." At their first performance, the audience was packed with more than 250 people. Word about the power of the chorus got out quickly, with help from local public radio, and at their next session the chorus grew from thirty-five members to seventy. By the end of the third fourteen-week session, the chorus had ninety people and decided to split into two groups. Jeanie saw it as good

Heder, Paul H

62441

Wednesday, September 23, 2020

31183198573799   Creative care : a revolut

timing—that the community was hungry for something positive and ambitious. "We are creative to our last breath," she said, "the one thing that keeps growing is our creativity. We just have to provide those experiences to each other." At latest count, the Giving Voice Chorus had more than 180 members, entirely supported by private donation. And the chorus's website and training tools have spawned at least twenty additional choruses across the country.

There are countless stories of the power of Giving Voice for its participants, care partners, volunteers, and elders alike. But the effects have been trickier to research. One study on the group found improvements in depression and quality of life for both people with dementia and their care partners. But the number in the study was so small (fewer than twenty people) that it is impossible to generalize the results.[3] There is a robust and growing community choir network across the world. Research on those choirs suggests that for older people (not necessarily those with dementia), community choirs promote social connections and increase happiness and self-esteem, while decreasing depression and anxiety.[4] One of the most robust studies was spearheaded by University of California, San Francisco's Dr. Julene Johnson, who led a three-year, randomized control study of twelve senior center choirs with a total of 390 singers. The choirs were led by professional directors and accompanists, met for ninety minutes each week, and gave several public performances, although less formal than Giving Voice's elaborate *Love Never Forgets*. The eagerly awaited results were that after six months, choir members reported being less lonely and more interested in life. But, disappointingly, researchers did not find improvements in physical or cognitive health.[5]

The dream is to get data showing that choirs improve our health or, even better, also reduce health-care costs. But while we wait for researchers to design large-scale studies and for funders to support them, let's not deny the power of experiencing those magic elements— what Kivnick identifies as "growth and mastery, being helpful and being helped." Participants share stories with Mary and Jeanie about Giving Voice giving them a reason to hope, a reason to get out of bed in the morning, and a way to share in something joyful with their care partner. But Mary says that at its heart, Giving Voice, like On a Positive Note, is about changing the stigma by changing expectations.

Mary was on stage with the chorus at the Ordway. "I was overwhelmed with their accomplishment singing nine new songs," she said. But the medical field, which is perhaps the most powerful authority for families with dementia, is hobbled by low expectations or perhaps more generously a general lack of awareness that the arts in general, and choral singing in particular, are even possibilities. Mary told me that the group recently sang at a major dementia conference in the Midwest. The chorus was sitting on stage nearby as two doctors were asked about what people with dementia can do to live well after diagnosis. "And they said, 'Eat well and exercise,'" said Mary. "It was stunning how they were not aware that there were sixty people sitting right there who were totally engaged and living well with Alzheimer's. It just didn't fit into their spiel."

A Beautiful Tenor

Three years later I drive the same highway back up to Appleton to On a Positive Note's Christmas concert. This time I don't even try to bribe the kids. They are swept away by school, sports, and their own concerts. It's just me walking into the concert, which is tucked in a small auditorium in the Building for Kids children's museum. This time, I carry with me the new and uneasy knowledge of my mother's official diagnosis of probable Alzheimer's. Actually, the latest diagnosis is the awkward and frightening-sounding major neurocognitive disorder of the Alzheimer's type. It's a weighty thing to carry with me into this buoyant room, where chorus members are wearing halos, reindeer antlers, and elf ears.

Mom loves choirs. She wrote family histories that always seemed to include mention of the "delightful Irish tenor" of an uncle or great grandfather. Her own grandparents had met when, exhausted and bewildered, her grandfather stepped off a long-haul train in Livingston, Montana. Without a sense of where he would sleep, he followed the angelic voices of a choir to the doors of the nearby church. He would later marry Kate Davis, one of the singers—no doubt a lovely Welsh tenor. I think of them as I watch the twenty-five or more choir members make their way through a parcel of traditional holiday songs. They have a professional choir director and a young accompanist, a piano major from the Lawrence University Conservatory, whom they clearly adore. Susan McFadden told me that at one of the rehearsals the singers asked if they could gather around him just so they could watch his hands move. The room is happy.

Bob is a robust gentleman with a Santa-like belly. He is wearing reindeer antlers. I can't tell whether he has dementia, is a caregiver, or is a volunteer, and it doesn't matter. He fills his lungs with air and the room with his resonant baritone. His face is relaxed. There is awe around the edges of his mouth and in his eyes, as they narrow with concentration. Singing with joy and confidence, he demands figgy pudding. He dreams of a white Christmas. He tells the tale of Frosty the Snowman. On a Positive Note is a hybrid. It is part sing-along, part elevated expectation (as evidenced by the choice to sing "Silent Night" in German), and all compassion and welcoming. Three women who were in the chorus that my son Ben photographed at the Congregational Church in 2016 are now widows, but they are still singing. Three members of a barbershop quartet volunteer to lend harmony. I think I can pick them out, but I'm not totally sure. There are adult children with their children in the audience with me, watching Grandma, or possibly Great-Grandma, having fun, making something beautiful, and belonging.

Sitting in that auditorium filled with Christmas music, I am hit with a memory of driving along a small country road in France. It is summer, and in my memory, the landscape is a dense tangle of green with tall narrow trees lining the roadside. But that might be from an image from a long-ago postcard collection. My parents had taken my college-aged sister and me to France for the wedding of longtime family friends. To pass the time as we drove south, my sister and I sang in the back seat. Silly old camp songs, or new folk tunes that we both had memorized. We knew my mom loved this. But, for whatever unexplainable reason, when she asked to join us, we tortured her by refusing to sing anymore. I hope that one of the blessings of dementia will be that she might forget that cruelty. And I vow to try my best to play and sing with her—without crying. I'm deeply thankful that my boys agreed to go with me on that Sunday afternoon in 2016. I don't much care about the research at this moment. I simply hope that if this journey catches me in it one day, my boys will remember how much I love to sing.

CHAPTER 14

"Wait, You *Live* Here?"

I f you had peered through the giant windows of the University of Wisconsin–Milwaukee's Kenilworth Gallery in June 2018, you would have seen Molly and Charlie, two undergraduate art majors, hovering around the food table, nervously rearranging the cups and napkins, the iced tea and lemonade. Molly is a fiber artist with gauges in her ears and snappy 1950s-style tortoiseshell glasses. Charlie is a jewelry major with a bold, short shock of blonde hair. The two had been working on this exhibit for months, and it was finally happening. Invitations were out. Artwork had been gathered and hung. Posters had been designed, printed, and taped in elevators at senior living communities on Milwaukee's east side and in the windows of local merchants by a team of elders at Eastcastle Place. This was the Flourish Fest, an annual exhibit featuring a year's worth of collaborative work of elders and art students from the University of Wisconsin–Milwaukee.

Molly and Charlie had a lot to be nervous about. The gallery is on a busy one-way street, and the shuttles from the care homes were pulling over on the opposite side, leading to a nerve-racking parade of people with walkers, canes, and wheelchairs in the middle of a block in a city where drivers do not believe in stopping for pedestrians. But gradually, and without incident, the elders made their way up the ramp into the gallery space and into the embrace of an arts student. Christina, a senior who had graduated just a few weeks earlier, welcomed her friends and neighbors from Ovation Chai Point, where she had been living for the past year, designing and offering arts programming in exchange for room and board as part of the Student Artist in Residence (SAIR) program. "The last thing I expected to be doing in my senior year of college was to be living in a senior living community," Christina said.

I don't know that I could have done what Christina did when I was in college. Even though I loved visiting my grandmother and her friends, I went home at the end of the day. The pacing and orientation of my days were still fast and dominated by youth. But with projects like Penelope and Islands of Milwaukee, I observed firsthand the budding connections between the elders and students—connections that ended abruptly when grades were posted for the semester. Even if students genuinely wanted to maintain the relationships, winter break at home or summer jobs got in the way. The SAIR program was born out of the hope that the longer a student stayed engaged with an elder community, the deeper the learning and relationships would be on both sides of what, in the United States, has become a cavernous generational divide.

Ageism and negative stereotypes of living beyond midlife are ubiquitous and stubborn, like stains so worn into the fabric of culture that we don't notice them anymore. Negative views of aging undergird inequities in nearly every corner of our lives, from career paths and the workplace, to housing, medical care, media representations, and educational systems. And their impact on individual health and well-being can be profound. Researchers have shown that people with negative views of aging live 7.5 years less than those with neutral or positive views of aging.[1] Other studies have shown when older adults are prompted with negative stereotypes about aging, they perform poorly on tests of working and episodic memory—that crucial form of memory that helps us order our own autobiography in time.[2]

Those who work in the field of aging care across the world have been crying foul for years. They see what's coming. There will be an enormous gap between the staffing needed to serve the growing aging population and the numbers of people who pursue studies in these fields—from clinical practitioners (dentists, nurses, doctors, social workers) to administrators and frontline staff doing the crucial work of tending to daily physical needs and nurturing emotional well-being. To recruit new staff, the aging care field must fight both low pay and the assumption that working with older adults is depressing and devoid of the satisfaction of a "cure." In the United States, market forces clearly aren't working when scores of geriatricians are needed to serve a burgeoning population, yet are remarkably scarce and earn roughly half as much as a cardiologist.[3]

Social media is not helping. Although the age demographics of Facebook are trending upward, a study in 2014 analyzed eighty-four groups on Facebook with a mean age of twenty-nine. They found that all but one focused on negative images of aging—ranging from what they called "excoriating" older adults (74 percent of the posts), to those that suggested banning older adults from daily activities such as shopping (a whopping 37 percent of posts).[4]

Research on ageism and its cultural impact has been growing slowly since Dr. Robert Butler coined the term "ageism" in 1969. A tale is emerging about the toll negative views on aging take on both the physical and the cognitive health of older adults, particularly in Western cultures. But what is the cost to young people? What is the cost of the implicit bias that forms from walking down the aisles of Walgreens or CVS, past the "age-killer," "anti-age" or "age-defying" lotions? Young people are future older people—if they are lucky. What happens when young people are barraged with negative images of aging, or experience an absence of images of or real-life relationships with older adults? What is the impact on young people's physical and cognitive health? Their career choices? The relationships in their lives—at home and in their communities? Does the negative view of aging affect young people's ability to imagine their future? To plan a meaningful life? To be supportive neighbors and citizens? Does ageism lead to reckless behavior? To narrowed career choices? Are the ageist cultural messages and infrastructures creating what Margaret Gullette calls "youth supremacists"?[5] And if so, how in heaven's name will they handle the changes time brings to their own bodies and minds?

Granted, this would be a tough study to carry out, seeing as it would mean following people across their entire lives. But there are little windows that offer a peek into the potential benefits of meaningful intergenerational relationships for young and old alike. Some of those windows are at the Kenilworth Gallery, where we can see into the culmination of a year of friendships formed through art-making between undergraduates and elders. In nearly every other chapter, my first concern is for the experience of the elders. My hope here is to focus on and share the stories and revelations of the student artists to illuminate a path toward more intergenerational friendships and ultimately, ideally, less ageism.

When the SAIR program first starts, new students commonly drag with them the residue of popular culture. They refer generically to "old people" and make awkward comparisons of working with elders to offering art programs for toddlers or children in elementary school. It was my job to encourage students to question these messages and to train them for the experiences that lay ahead. But how exactly does one prepare a twenty-year-old for a year of living in a care home? What does one say in advance, and what does one simply let the student discover? For most of the students, death has never been closer than the shadow of a distant great-uncle or great-grandparent. And frailty is a crisp blue-and-white icon of a person in a wheelchair relegated to parking spots, bus seats, and bathroom stalls. How does one prepare the students for a shift in the balance of silence and noise, of stillness and speed? How do I explain the folding over of time and memory? Or how someone long passed can be a vivid, everyday presence?

After several years of trial and error, the care staff, elder mentors, and I hit upon a delicate balance. First, we recruit students with promises of adventure, purpose, real-life job skills, and the sizeable savings of a year's room and board. Then we hold a group interview and try our best to scare students away. The mentors, program staff, and potential student artists in residence gather around a conference table, and we talk about some of the realities they will encounter: You'll make a plan for a workshop and find you have to toss the whole thing out the window because it won't work on that day. But you'll learn the incredible skill of improvising on the spot. Friends your own age might stop hanging out with you because they are uncomfortable with older people and cannot figure out why you are living among them. That's okay. Maybe those friends weren't really such great friends. You'll make new, older friends too. They will be amazingly supportive friends with deep life experience. But they might die or get sick while you're living there.

Some students drop out after the interview, and that is always the right choice for them. Some students are juggling eighteen credits and two jobs, and the added time commitment and emotional challenges will prove too much. The ones we don't manage to scare away move into the care homes with eyes and hearts open. To kick off their training, the program matches each student artist in residence with a staff mentor and an elder mentor to act as confidant, conscience, and reality check all in one. The mentors and student artists in residence attend a daylong retreat to learn engagement techniques and the basics of aging-care settings. Together the mentors and student artists in residence create their own code of ethics to guide their practice throughout the year. In Molly and Charlie's year, the SAIR code of ethics included the usual standards of being prepared and on time. But the code also included standards like these:

* Be flexible, patient, humble, and dependable.
* Create an infectious sense of fun and discovery.
* Express gratitude and graciousness.
* Don't underestimate the capacity of elders.
* Create time for just being present in people's lives.

Even after the opening retreat, nerves and uncertainty can run high. Erin, a quiet visual art major with a wide, warm smile, lived at Chai Point the year before Christina. She vividly remembered her move-in day. Her friends were all moving into their apartments. "My mom packed up the Subaru and we pulled up into the circle drive in front of Chai Point and I looked up and thought, 'Wow. I'm living here.'" It was an adjustment for the staff, too. "They kept asking me if I was helping my mom or grandmom," Erin told me. "No, I'm moving in," she explained.

But her very first day also gave Erin a sense of the generosity of her new community. Exhausted from moving, Erin had taken a short nap, and she woke up ravenous. "I was going to have sweet potato burritos but couldn't find a can opener." So she knocked on her neighbor's door, introduced herself, and asked if she could borrow a can opener. "She kind of looked a little off-put, so I was backing away, and she stopped me and said 'No, no—it's fine,' and she gave me her electric can opener," Erin said. When she was done, Erin returned the can opener. Her neighbor, who she learned was named Karen, was surprised to see it again. "She thought I wanted to keep it! No wonder she was put off. I couldn't believe this woman would give a total stranger her electric can opener!" It was the beginning of a beautiful friendship that continued after Erin moved out and traveled the world. "I Facetimed with her from Portugal," said Erin, smiling as she relived the memory.

It took Christina a while to adjust as well. "I remember in the beginning, it felt so weird to call Chai Point 'home,'" she wrote in her final reflections on the experience. "I would be on campus like 'Alright, time to go home!'" She would start walking toward her old apartment that she shared with friends, only to stop and remember "that my home now is actually a retirement home." But those feelings shifted gradually. "I now feel way more like a community member and neighbor," wrote Christina.

As the student artists in residence learned the daily rhythms of their new homes and began developing a following at their arts workshops, several talked about how nice it felt to have people worry over them. Erin rode her bike the two miles to campus each day, and her friends at Chai Point knew she was home if her bike was parked out front. "One night it was snowing pretty hard, so I left my bike on campus and took the bus," Erin told me. "It caused quite a panic! People were worried that I was lost in the snowstorm because my bike wasn't there."

The workshops the student artists in residence develop are focused primarily on building community, with some attention to growing artistic skill as well. I found their workshop ideas breathtaking in their creativity. Ian, who lived at Eastcastle Place for two years, held a T-shirt swap and an intergenerational game night. He invited his college friends to join his Eastcastle Place friends to exchange old shirts or teach one another Sheepshead, cribbage, or euchre. Molly did felt-soap workshops, button-making, and a community weaving to which everyone could contribute. Tania did a T-shirt printing workshop. I asked Erin about her favorite workshop, and she told me about Love Day. "That was definitely my favorite," she said. "I had a friend that played guitar, so he came, and we all painted rocks with hearts on them." They just did silly things, but they all had fun, and her studio was overflowing with people. "We wrote stories or just answered questions about love," she said. "I remember Helen, who lived down the hall from me, she told us that after being married for so long, she and her husband didn't give each other cards anymore for Valentine's Day. They just went to the drugstore rack and read them to each other."

Throughout the year, the student artists in residence have monthly check-ins with mentors and biweekly check-ins with one another as they navigate the emotional terrain of confronting their own fears and becoming part of their communities. "I'm so thankful for you all," said Thorin at a SAIR check-in. Thorin was an acting student living in Luther Manor's independent living apartments, known as the Terrace. Ever since the Penelope project, Luther Manor residents had been writing and staging original plays under the direction of Rusty Tym. They were eager for student artists in residence with theater chops. Thorin bonded quickly with his Luther Manor theater friends, but his same-aged friends were more of a challenge. "None of my friends understand my daily life now—it's so different from theirs. It's so helpful to come here and know that you get it."

In those biweekly meetings, the student artists in residence bonded over experiences like what they called the "Wait, you *live* here?" moment. Erin told of one encounter on the elevator when one of her neighbors observed that Erin was there an awful lot and that she must be very close to whomever it was she was visiting. "No," Erin told the neighbor, "I live here." The woman took a moment to take in the information and then, in a hushed, sympathetic tone, asked, "Is there something wrong with you?" "Oh, no," Erin explained with a smile. "I am here for you! I offer arts workshops for the community."

Thorin had been drawn to the SAIR program to share with elders what he had learned about the physical and emotional benefits of performance training. A severe back injury had haunted him for years until he found meditation and yoga. In his first month living in and learning about his new community at Luther Manor, Thorin shifted gears. He noticed that many of his neighbors already had established workout routines in their fitness room, but that they talked about wanting to write. So he created a weekly writing group. His following grew slowly over time. Several weeks in, the regulars were sharing poems and short stories of their lives. Thorin, well over six foot and with long, golden brown hair pulled back into a bun, thought it might be time for him to share his own writing. "So I started reading from an autobiographical piece I wrote a couple months ago. About halfway through, I realized that this story was pretty R-rated, and I blushed pretty badly." He blushed again, as he told us the story at our biweekly gathering of student artists in residence. "But," said Thorin smiling, "Joyce reached over and patted my knee and said, 'It's okay, honey, we've heard it all before—and then some.'"

Later that spring, Thorin's theater troupe lost its venue for a performance of *Richard III*. His Luther Manor friends reserved a space at the Terrace and welcomed the troupe with a full crowd. His Luther Manor friends also carpooled across town for Thorin's final matinee performance in his senior year. At the Flourish Fest that spring, Thorin invited his writing group; he displayed written versions of their stories and created recordings of them reading their stories aloud. Visitors listened intently on headphones to the stories his friends had honed over their weeks together. Midway through the afternoon program, the student artists in residence gathered to share their parting words with the elders, staff, and family from the SAIR sites. Usually a powerful stage presence, Thorin struggled to get through his prepared thank-you speech without choking up.

Molly was a student artist in residence for two years. In the beginning of her first year she struggled to figure out how to engage with elders. At one of our SAIR meetings, she put it this way: "I'm funny," she explained, with her usual deadpan delivery. "I'm a funny person. This is how my friends know me. It's how I know the world. But I don't know what's funny to an eighty-seven-year-old woman with Alzheimer's. How can I bond with people if I don't know what's funny to them?" It's a good question. Gradually, over Molly's two years of experience, first at St. John's on the Lake and then at Eastcastle Place, where she joined the choir and formed enduring friendships, Molly found her rhythm. Still, differences in generational humor could catch her off guard. One of her best friends at Eastcastle Place was a woman named Pat, who shared Molly's sharp wit. They were screen-printing small doodles that Molly had originally created as part of her senior thesis project. One of the doodles was a ring. Admiring the drawing, Pat told Molly she should open up a jewelry store when she grows up. "Then I asked her what she wanted to be when she grew up," wrote Molly, "and she promptly responded, 'In a casket!' I'm laughing right now just thinking about it."

At the end of their yearlong experience, the student artists in residence share final reflections on what they learned. The themes have been consistent across the four years the program has been evolving: student artists in residence learn patience, empathy, how to engage people with disabilities in art-making, and how to approach aging and frailty in their own families and lives. Tania was a student artist in residence at St. John's on the Lake working with people with memory loss as well as those in their independent apartments—a handful of whom had been professional artists. For Tania, the experience helped her process her own challenging relationships with her *abuelo* and *abuela*, who had raised her. Through her experiences with the elders at St. John's, Tania said she was able to see them as people with different life experiences and expectations—not just demanding grandparents. "For this, and for the healing it helped me have with my abuela before her passing, I will be forever grateful for being part of this beautiful program," wrote Tania.

Christina always thought of herself as a patient and easygoing person. But her experience at Chai Point put this patience to the test in a very specific place—at the elevator. With all the walkers, wheel-chairs, and canes, and the general snail's pace of walking and life in a care community, doing something that normally took Christina a few seconds could take what seemed like forever. Older people, she observed, needed time "to mentally register that the elevator has ar-rived and then needed more time to get inside." In the beginning this pace drove her crazy. But gradually, she came to see time quite differ-ently. "Moments like this help remind me that time truly is a man-made concept and that I really never need to be rushing around quite as much as I think. I have come to realize that having a rushed feel-ing about you can come off as abrasive to some, and that taking a couple extra minutes in certain cases can help communicate respect," she wrote.

Christina had other realizations as well, particularly about people with memory loss. She described herself as wanting people to "get to the point" of everything and having to fight that wiring within her-self in her daily encounters at Chai Point. She would get anxious and annoyed when Sarah would tell the same long story about being a schoolteacher. But then Christina came to realize that her frustration said more about her than about Sarah and "does literally nothing for either of us" in that moment: "Of course, Sarah doesn't realize that she's told me this story so many times." That story was a strong part of Sarah's identity, and Christina realized that there was something in the story that was important for Sarah to share: "I have learned to really pay attention to what is repeated by those with memory loss because . . . these stories reveal which memories mean the most to them, and it helps me ask better questions in response."

Could I have articulated that understanding so clearly at her age? As I walked down the nursing home hallway to see my grandmother? As the rhythmic cries of "Help me" floated by on stale air? My hindsight observations are dramatically improved with progressive lenses. But these college juniors and seniors are negotiating tough entanglements of gender, age, race, and physical and cognitive abilities. The students are confronting their own fears over a full academic year—not just in the classroom, but where the students eat, sleep, and find solace. And they are emerging with insights beyond their years—insights that I am learning from and that I think anyone living and working with elders in any setting can benefit from.

In the year that Molly and Christina were curating the Flourish Fest, I had asked them to invite SAIRs to include snippets from their journals and reflections in the exhibits themselves, so that their observations would appear side-by-side with the elders' artwork that emerged in the workshops over the year. Erin wrote hers directly on the wall. One featured a picture and four pieces of advice from her friend Thelma:

1. "Don't spend your time with a bully."

2. "Find the best catch."

3. "Even through the crummy days, look at the good things you've been given. *That* is what matters."

4. "I love you too, now go do your homework."

Molly and Charlie helped Tania put a dozen excerpts from her journal on the gallery walls. In one, she wrote, "I had not realized just how much our society evades speaking about the last big period of our lives. No one likes to think about aging. Hence, no one speaks about it all." In another she wrote: "The act of art making and creating art in collaborative form propels deeper rooted talk and sharing. This exchange is what drives me."

Molly has now graduated and is running the SAIR program as the administrator. She has dreams of expanding the Flourish Fest into a citywide festival and collaborating with TimeSlips to spread the program across the country. Only by disrupting the age segregation that goes unnoticed for both college students and older people can they truly learn with and from each other. Some of the students applied to the program on a lark, lured in by the idea of free room and board. None of them has said it was easy. But all of them said they would do it again. Christina described the program as "one of the most random, serendipitous moments of my life so far and it will be something that I will hold dear to my heart for the rest of my life." Just to make sure their reflections weren't simply sweetened for a better grade, I sent out an anonymous survey to all those who had gone through the program over the previous four years. One response captured it all: "This was the most challenging, difficult and beautiful experience I have gone through. I would do it again in a blink of an eye."

Throughout the year, relationships form, and stereotyped notions of aging begin to fall away. When the students arrange to host a workshop, they post flyers on bulletin boards and cross their fingers that someone shows up. And the elders who do show up, week after week, do so as much to support the nervous students as to take the opportunity to learn and grow through drawing or writing, through dancing or painting. These are not just generic "old people" anymore. These are the students' friends.

What if the SAIR program experience was normal?

What if senior housing units reserved apartments for young people in college or emerging into the workforce?

What if we all understood that taking your time is a sign of respect?

What if care settings realized that they could hire artists to enrich the daily life of their communities?

What if I could have done this at their age?

CHAPTER 15

"I'm Worth Stopping For"

In my ride-alongs with Meals on Wheels delivery drivers, I observed something that haunted me. I noticed that as I followed Mr. Johnny in his pickup truck, we pulled up to apartment building after apartment building that was directly across the street from a grocery store—or, in some cases, an entire block of restaurants and stores. There were affordable food sources not a hundred yards away from the doorsteps of elders who were receiving three or four Meals on Wheels deliveries each week. But I also observed that the cars on those four- and six-lane streets that separated the apartment buildings from the stores and restaurants were going forty miles an hour, if not faster. I was scared to cross that street in the time the lights allowed. I couldn't imagine some of the people I saw answering the door to accept their meals making it ten feet before horns blasted and the noses of cars pushed forward to bully them into speeding up their crossing.

Inspired by this observation, one of the Questions of the Day that was delivered with the meals was, "Is there an intersection you wish you could cross on foot, but feel it's too dangerous?" We were flooded with responses. Some handwritten cards collected and returned by the drivers listed five intersections. One woman called the project's voice-mail line to share her panic. She lived at a busy intersection across from a church. She couldn't bear to look out her living room window anymore for fear that one of the elders would be hit as they crossed to attend services. For Milwaukee drivers, like so many drivers across the United States, pedestrians are an afterthought, an inconvenient intrusion to their right of way.

What if frail elders could be invited into making meaningful and lasting change in their communities?

Surely frailty does not preclude interest in or capacity for activism—for shaping the world they will leave behind?

Within weeks, I was sitting around a table at the Kelly Senior Center with Bob Pietrykowski and Debby Pizur, the humble and tenacious leaders of a senior advocacy group that was committed to the issue of pedestrian safety. The little group with the big name— South Shore Connecting Caring Communities—was a formidable committee made up of neighborhood retirees and leaders from area service agencies. Elders in the communities they served were scared by recent deadly crashes, one of which had left an elder dying in the street with no cars stopping to aid him. Bob complained that they had been having trouble getting their local alderman to take the issue seriously. They told me he brushed them off, saying, "I can either stop the people who don't stop for pedestrians or I can stop the violent criminals. What's your choice?" I told Bob and Debby that I thought

our efforts could amplify theirs—that we might be able to use performance to help get the alderman's attention. Based on their experience
and the map we had put together from the hundreds of responses
from the Question of the Day card, we identified three intersections
on which we would concentrate our efforts.

Working together with Sojourn Theatre and students from the
UWM Theatre Department, our team jumped into the research. It
turns out that elders and children are the most vulnerable pedestrians. In 2017 in the United States, 5,984 pedestrians died in crashes,
a 27 percent increase since 2007.[1] Of those, 19 percent were older
adults and 21 percent were children,[2] a sad but strong argument for
cross-generational advocacy. The increase in pedestrian deaths has
myriad causes; perhaps most notably, this is the decade that cell
phones became ubiquitous, driver education classes disappeared from
public schools, and marijuana became legal in several states. Larger
cars with higher bumpers also became more popular—and more
deadly for pedestrians. Research tells us that the difference between
a car hitting you at twenty miles an hour versus thirty-five miles an
hour is likely the difference between an injury and death.[3]

The UWM Theatre students and I went to the three intersections
the South Shore Connecting Caring Communities group had identified. We brought tape measures, pens, and a giant sketch pad. We
walked the area to get a feel for it. We drew maps. We timed the
lights. We measured the distances. We took note of damaged sidewalks. We looked for senior apartment buildings and schools nearby.
We asked building managers if they'd be interested in hosting a
workshop that we playfully called "How to Stop Traffic: Empowering
Pedestrians." We learned that at one of the intersections we selected

there were five senior apartment buildings within two hundred yards and a grocery store and pharmacy on the corner. All five apartment buildings had vans to drive the elders to the store because it was too dangerous for them to navigate the intersection.

At another of the intersections we selected, a senior apartment building towered across the street from two schools. Twice a day, a crossing guard helped pedestrians across the street. Still, the police in this small suburban municipality of St. Francis sent an officer every day because they were worried that drivers would ignore the guard. When the theater students and I visited that intersection to map and measure what would become our route, we struck up a conversation with a woman who was excited to join us on the day of the performances. She often took the bus downtown and was nervous every time she had to get to the bus stop across the street. "We'll get you across safely," the students assured her. "Good," she said, "I have a doctor's appointment that day!"

In our research, we found David Engwicht, an Australian "creative placemaker" and activist whose mission was to make roads safer for cyclists and pedestrians. His approach? Appeal to the human being inside the driver.[4] Engwicht believes that using humor and compelling stories can intrigue drivers, interrupting their urgency and aggressiveness, and enticing them to slow down. His early work in reclaiming streets was based on data that showed that street speed was related to how much pedestrians had retreated from walking. This was exactly what Bob and Debby had observed in their neighborhoods. The elders had stopped trying to cross.

We also learned that on the other side of the world, the upstart mayor of Bogotá, Colombia, Antanas Mockus, was using a similar approach. To tame the unruly streets of Bogotá, which had one of the worst crash rates in South America, Mockus hired 420 street mimes to shame and ridicule those who ignored the laws: drivers and pedestrians alike. Known for his unorthodox approach to governing, Mockus describes his philosophy this way: "Knowledge empowers people. If people know the rules, and are sensitized by art, humor, and creativity, they are much more likely to accept change."[5] The approach worked. Traffic deaths dropped by half during his tenure. Inspired by Engwicht's and Mockus's approaches, our team set about creating a story for a street performance that would intrigue not only drivers, but also civic officials who seemed tone deaf to how urgent this issue is for so many of their elder constituents.

What would our story be? In Milwaukee, a band of street mimes mocking drivers would likely end with dead street mimes. Our story would need to draw on our own cultural roots. What characters might intrigue drivers enough to compel them to stop or slow down? What story would be so clear that it could be communicated in the twenty seconds (or less in some cases) that the lights give pedestrians to cross? To find a story that resonated locally, we did workshops at senior apartment buildings and senior living communities. There were a wide range of elders—from those who were just a little unsteady on their feet to those riding wheelchairs, from those with no significant cognitive challenges to those who struggled to take in the beautiful questions we asked. "What is the dialogue between drivers and pedestrians?" I asked. I got lots of raised middle fingers and blue shades of shouting. It didn't matter what the pedestrians said, many told me. The drivers' windows are closed, and pedestrians feel powerless against the car. "Well, what would you say to a driver if you could?" I pressed. Again, there were some blue responses of revenge and frustration. But one woman, in the workshop at Ovation Chai Point, leaned forward in her wheelchair, and looked right into the camera of my phone as I recorded her response. She said firmly and slowly, in a thin voice, "It's simple. I'm worth stopping for."

And so the motto of the project was born: "We're worth stopping for."

The story itself emerged from brainstorming about when and why cars willingly stop. Milwaukee is perched on Lake Michigan, but it is also crosscut by three rivers. In the heart of downtown, it is common to hear a clanging alarm and see a flashing red light and a large red-and-white-striped safety arm drop down across the road before the bridge is raised and a tall-masted boat makes its way down the river. The protocol is drilled into drivers. If you hear the clanging, you know you must stop. You can't edge into the intersection. You can't turn left or right, or you'll end up in the water. You just stop. And wait. This would be the perfect narrative. Together, the theater students, Sojourn actors, and anyone else who showed up to cross with us that day—we would become that safety arm and those guardrails. We would embody that tall-masted boat. And the drivers would stop—we hoped.

Sojourn Theatre's designer Shannon Scrofano went to work. She created drawings of a whole ship's worth of sails: a giant square topsail for which she fashioned a belt-like holster; a trapezoid-shaped "standing lug" sail; a simple triangle sail; and a whole series of smaller, brightly colored sails that could be used as walking sticks for older performers. The topsail was so large that we worried that a gust of wind might carry away our actor. With the new storyline in place, I wrote letters to civic officials at each of the three municipalities in which we would be performing. I invited the mayors of Milwaukee, St. Francis, and Cudahy. I invited the county supervisors. I invited the aldermen. I invited the state senators. "Join us for a performance designed to teach drivers to see and stop for pedestrians," I wrote, adding that we were inviting the media and would have a "media stop" in the performance for the politicians to explain their stance on safe, walkable, and healthy cities for all citizens. Nothing could make the case for lengthening the lights and enforcing the existing laws like a mayor and an elder constituent stuck in the middle of an intersection. It was an election year. I crossed my fingers and mailed the letters.

No performance like this had been tried in Milwaukee. Without a precedent, I wanted to make sure that all three municipalities would be supportive of our merry band of street crossers—or at least that the police would not ticket us. So I called the community liaison at each of the three police stations. I researched whether we might need some kind of permit. Our plan was to cross during the lights, so we were not going to impede traffic. We didn't need to hood any meters. We were not going to block sidewalks. We were just walking. It didn't seem like we needed a permit to do that. But still unsure, I called the City of Milwaukee's permit office and explained our situation. The woman at the desk that day listened intently. "It's your God-given right to cross the street, honey," she told me confidently. "You don't need a permit." And then she thanked me for the project. "I have multiple sclerosis," she explained. She felt that hot swell of fear that comes with staring down impatient drivers every day.

The plans were set. Each performance would last two hours. We would gather in a friendly starting spot (a church or nearby apartment building) and head out to the intersection. A Sojourn performer played the Ship Captain, complete with hat and megaphone to inspire his crew. We gathered a playlist of every song about the sea or sailing that we could think of, including the theme songs to *The Love Boat* and *Gilligan's Island*. The stage manager would always be the last one to cross the street in case there was any trouble. The theater students played the parts of the alarm (ringing triangles) and the guardrails (carrying a ten-foot piece of white plastic pipe marked with red stripes) and carried signs. During the rehearsals in intersections near the UWM campus, we were nearly struck by a car whose driver mindlessly turned right and directly into our group crossing the street. The plastic pipe guardrail literally saved our lives. We realized that we needed large, visible signs to give advance warning of the performance to drivers, to let them know how long it would last, and to reward good behavior. The signs read, "AHOY! PERFORMANCE AHEAD!" "THANK YOU FOR SEEING AND STOPPING FOR PEDESTRIANS!" and "THIS PERFORMANCE WILL END IN 20 SECONDS!" Guardrails went first, followed by the triangles, then the "boat" (the captain and all those carrying sails) would cross.

We printed posters and put them up in storefronts, schools, and apartment buildings surrounding all three intersections. We sent press releases to all the papers and television stations, but just in case no one took the bait we also hired our own video crew to follow us. Volunteers had a range of options: They could play triangles. They could hold signs. They could walk with a sail and become part of the boat. They could hand out programs to interested onlookers and irritated or confused drivers. During the welcome gathering, director Maureen Towey encouraged people to think of this as "the most fun they would ever have crossing the street."

The day of the performance, May 1, was a classic blustery midwestern spring day: misty and cold in a bone-chilling, can't-get-warm kind of way. We would perform in Milwaukee's Bayview neighborhood that afternoon (before rush hour) and in the two suburban locations the following day. We had invited all the elders from the neighborhood workshops: the students from nearby schools, civic officials, stakeholders vested in pedestrian safety like the city engineers and the dean of UWM's new School of Public Health. Would anyone show up on a day like this?

Staff from the Church of the Immaculate Conception welcomed us and generously opened the front doors to let us gather out of the sting of the rain. Then miraculously, the weather improved. The dean of the School of Public Health was the first to show. "Just tell me how I can be helpful," she said eagerly. "I'm here for you." Slowly, a crowd grew. The ladies from the church grabbed a couple of sails. The adorable four-year-old son of a colleague from UWM joyfully took up one of the extra triangles. Sojourn performer James Hart gave a hearty captain's bellow: "Welcome aboard mates!" The mayor of Milwaukee arrived, followed by the heads of various programs in the County Department on Aging, the county supervisor, and the state senator. Someone running for state assembly showed too. A group of students with special needs from the nearby intermediate school gathered at the corner and eagerly awaited the show. The local art critic arrived with a colleague from Madison in tow. Several city specialists in planning and engineering joined us. And out of the corner of my eye I spotted the elusive alderman. He didn't join the performance, but he watched attentively.

Then Angie arrived. Angie is a force. She had answered every single Question of the Day delivered by her Meals on Wheels driver to her small apartment in St. Francis. It was hard for her to write, so she left detailed responses on our voice-mail line. She and our project assistant Chelsea created finger paintings together. Still, Angie was eager for more, so Chelsea asked Angie whether she could write a poem about crossing the street. And she did, calling it "A Stroker Crossing Over." "It's about me," Angie told us. "It's about crossing over—in more ways than one." Angie used a wheelchair, propelling herself forward with her feet. One hand, immobile and tightly clutched in a fist, rested in her lap. When she arrived with a caregiver and a couple of Chelsea's friends who had helped with transportation, Angie got right to work. "You must be the mayor," she said, and soon she had the dean of the School of Public Health and the mayor bending to listen to Angie's ideas on making the streets safer for pedestrians of all ages.

When we started the actual crossing part of the performance, I was giddy. Captain James had us lined up on the edge of the intersection. Jake, a theater student who had rehearsed with the giant sail, steadied it with a wide stance against any bursts of wind. When the light changed, the students carrying the guardrails comically highstepped into the intersection with a "Hup! Hup! Hup!" and poles straight up in the air. As the triangle ringers stepped forward, the guardrails slowly lowered to an official-looking horizontal position. Then into the intersection stepped the boat, with an array of sails waving in the wind. The captain led us in a simple sea shanty we had just practiced in the church lobby. The drivers seemed perplexed— just as Engwicht or Mockus would have hoped. And as if to anticipate their confusion, the sign holders playfully wiggled their three-foot, boldly lettered signs toward the drivers: "Thank you for

SEEING and STOPPING for pedestrians!" The sail holders offered friendly waves and echoed the signs' message: "Thank you!" The stage manager, noticing the timing of the lights, hurried us across, and the last sail holder stepped up onto the curb as the guardrails "Hup-hupped" out of the street and onto the curb behind us. All twenty of us made it across in time, including Angie, who had to pull herself over a few extra feet to find a curb cut.

We crossed all around the crazy triangle intersection at Kinnick-innic, Logan, and Russell Avenues with sails, signs, poles, and triangles. We crossed at stoplights with a hurried pace dictated by short lights, and at stop signs where we could chat and cross at our leisure. We sang along to Christopher Cross's "Sailing." The intermediate school students cheered us on. Cars honked—some out of irritation, some in a sign of support. Either way, the sign holders would break into broad grins and wiggle their signs in their direction. After one full round of crossing, we assembled back on the steps of the Church of the Immaculate Conception and, in my admiral role, I invited the mayor, the dean, the county supervisor, and the state senator to the center of the stairs. In a V formation around them, the theater students gathered and shared the words of the elders we had heard from in the workshops over the past several months. The brief performance ended with all of them saying in unison, "We're worth stopping for." I'd like to remember everyone cheering, but I think it was too cold for that. And for the local news film crew as well, who left after the first few crossings. But our own film crew captured the event, along with the civic officials' sharing their commitment to improving pedestrian safety.

The weather wasn't much better the next day, but our spirits were high. Our first stop was St. Francis. The police greeted us. Just as with the school crossing guard, they didn't want us crossing alone. I asked them to watch from the sidewalk—or better yet cross with us—unless they thought it was absolutely necessary to jump in and direct traffic. At this crossing, a busload of elders from an area care home arrived to cross with us. We slowed the boat to make sure we all made it across in time. The mayor of St. Francis arrived just in time for the media stop. As she was making her remarks, our friend who had the doctor's appointment stepped out of the door of the apartment building and crossed in the middle of the block, directly to the bus stop on the other side. She didn't walk to the corner and risk that a driver would blow through the sign into a right turn on red. Even with us there to usher her across, she knew what we had learned in research—that crossing at the corner put one at significantly higher risk of injury or death. I told the mayor, "I think we have our solution to that menacing right turn. Put the crosswalk right there!"

The last crossing site, a classic suburban street in Cudahy, was the most powerful experience of all three. We gathered at one of the five senior apartment buildings just down from the corner, and many of the people I had met at the workshop a month earlier came out to cross with us. Nancy, with tightly coiffed, bright white hair, used a walker. Lois used a scarf to protect her hair from the wind and grabbed a sail to use as a walking stick on our journey to the intersection. The mayor of Cudahy, a friendly man in his mid-fifties, arrived early and walked side by side with Nancy as she navigated the railroad tracks on the way to the corner. At the intersection, the mayor jokingly took a stance like a sprinter preparing to run a race. James called, "All ahead full!" and the guardrails and triangles burst into the street. The mayor and Nancy made it about halfway across when the director realized they wouldn't make it in time. A big green pickup truck revved its engine and inched forward, signaling his eagerness to make the left-hand turn. "Signs!" yelled the director, and the signs surrounded the stragglers on the boat, hoping to diffuse the driver's aggression with humor. The signs worked. We made it across. But the mayor and Nancy were rattled. Robert Schneider, the UWM urban planning expert who had been observing the performance, explained why. "These lights are substandard," he said. "They are supposed to be a second for every three feet. These are short by at least five seconds."[6]

We took stock. Everyone was okay, but it was a rough first crossing. The others proved easier, and the staff at the oil change shop on the corner offered friendly waves and cheers of support. When we arrived at the grocery store, the students gave their brief performance, and I invited the civic officials up to make their statements. The mayor was humbled by the experience. He promised action to help Nancy and Lois get safely to the store. As we prepared to head back, someone from the grocery store approached with a box of cookies. "These are from the guys across the street," she said. The oil change guys had bought us treats.

A few weeks later, I was back at the conference table at the Kelly Senior Center with Bob and Debby to compare notes and assess the impact of the project. Debby told me that the mayor of Cudahy had made sure that the lights were lengthened the very next week and that he was putting in place a longer-term assessment of that intersection with the city engineer. Bob said that in the Bayview neighborhood, the alderman had instituted a "sting" operation with the police. They were giving warnings for minor infractions and tickets for major ones. A big digital sign greeted people in both directions in advance of the intersection: "Slow down! Pedestrians are worth stopping for." The elders had made real change in their communities. James and I shared what we learned in Milwaukee with the Age-Friendly Pittsburgh initiative, which in turn staged several Crossings in that city. The elders' ideas and experiences rippled outward to affect the lives of people of all ages across the country.

What other changes could elders make? Why do so many people assume older people are only interested in or capable of sharing memories and stories of their experiences? While these are certainly valuable, the impulse to harvest the stories of elders rests on the notion that they are no longer interested in or capable of engaging in the world around them, or in making changes to the world they will leave behind. Perhaps there is also an assumption that politics is best left out of care settings. But working toward social and community change doesn't need to divide us. Instead it can be the very thing that brings people together, out of isolation and into purpose and belonging.

A Stroker Crossing Over
By Angie Tesch

One foot out, you hear a rumble and a roar.
You don't want to be a blob of gore,
So one foot back for the speed you lack.
One foot out and the other foot out,
You hear a roar.
Oh, what a bore.
You look to the right—the traffic is coming

Oh no, not again.

You move back with all your might.

You look to the left—more traffic is coming.

You look all around

Hoping to cross over to the park before dark

This would be such a lark.

CHAPTER 16

Wendy's Neverland, or Can Creative Care Be Scaled?

> Of course the Neverlands vary a good deal. John's, for instance, had a lagoon with flamingos flying over it at which John was shooting, while Michael, who was very small, had a flamingo with lagoons flying over it. John lived in a boat turned upside down on the sands, Michael in a wigwam, Wendy in a house of leaves deftly sewn together.
>
> **J. M. BARRIE,**
> *Peter Pan*

> *Never* put me in a nursing home.
>
> **EVERYONE, EVERYWHERE, ALWAYS**

I first heard from the force of nature who is Angie McAllister in 2012. She had the best job title I could imagine. She was director of cultural transformation for sixty of Signature HealthCARE's rural nursing homes. Angie had heard of the Penelope project and emailed me asking whether I had thought of replicating it in other homes. Of course I had. The way to truly transform care would be to get creative care practices into every care setting—but how?

A thorough evaluation of the Penelope project had confirmed our instincts about which elements of the project were crucial to building a strong sense of community.[1] The TimeSlips team had just begun folding those lessons into our training on a large scale, teaching the core elements of creative care and walking staff through the planning of celebration events. In essence, we were infusing the creative process into the daily rhythms of care systems. We trained staff at fifty nursing homes across the State of Wisconsin and held a joint celebration at the Alzheimer's Association Wisconsin State Conference. Together, some nine hundred conference attendees danced and sang to animations that featured elders reading the stories they had written and choreographed. The energy in the room was through the roof. My face hurt from smiling. Talk about awe.

The conference session was fun, but the real magic would be to stage a work of art inside the homes themselves. The real magic would be to go beyond "activities" to inviting family and neighbors to experience the care setting as a place of possibility, not just illness and death. To experience care itself as an opportunity for shared creation.

I genuinely wasn't sure whether the deep magic of the Penelope project could be replicated across multiple homes. Health systems are rigid. Nursing homes in particular are highly regulated. Turnover is commonplace. If you managed to infuse wonder and responsiveness into such a system, if just one or two people leave or resist, old patterns can take over again. If we were to replicate a Penelope-like project in multiple homes, such an effort would need to evolve over time, anticipate turnover, and allow for a gradual seeping in of the power of creative care. Such a project would tackle an epic story, a story older than the oldest person in the room, one that everyone already felt they knew in a subconscious way. Such a project would turn outward, inviting family and volunteers to engage as equals with the elders. It would be accessible and inclusive of people of all abilities. It would unfold organically, not evolving from a preconceived plan but building on the input of all those who came to the table. Such a project would partner with artists—not as dictators of an artistic vision but as equal collaborators in discovering the work. It would take a giant, bold leap beyond bingo and balloon toss. Beyond even sing-alongs and computer games. It would create beauty. It would create legacy, meaning, and joy. It would transform the care setting from a stigmatized health center into a vibrant cultural center.

That is a big, bold dream.

The more I got to know Angie, the more I realized that if such a dream could be realized, she was the one who could help make it happen, compelled by the sheer force of her will and her bedrock belief in the dignity of every human being. Born and raised in Kentucky, Angie was awarded a rare full-ride scholarship to college, only to quit school to fulfill what she felt was a calling to work with elders. Her parents scratched their heads as she dropped out and became a certified nursing assistant. Pretty quickly, her supervisors realized that Angie had a unique vision and the capacity to fulfill it. She became a "restorative aide," then an activity director. She arrived at Signature HealthCARE in 2007 as a quality-of-life director with some very clear ideas about what needed to change in nursing homes.[2] "It started with this very frail gentleman who asked me if I could help him fulfill his dream of going to Savannah, Georgia, to see his squadron honored in an Air Force Museum there," she told me. "Well, I sure wasn't gonna say no to him." She made it happen. Some eleven years later, Signature now takes groups of elders on some twenty vacations every year. Elders bring wheelchairs to the beach or take in the sights at Disney World, a game at Fenway Park, or a Broadway show in New York City. When Angie dreamed of bringing children into the nursing homes, she created a summer camp for the children of staff. She started with one. Signature now has summer camps at sixty of its homes.

So Angie and I set to it. We shared dreams and visions of a story that built on the intergenerational foundation of her summer camps. We looked at maps. We drove long hours across the hills of Kentucky visiting homes. We considered funding. We looked for artists with a range of skills (music, theater, visual) who lived near the rural nursing homes and national artists who could inspire a vision across all the participating homes. And we looked for an evaluation team who could track our progress. One year and twenty-seven drafts of a grant proposal later, we were funded to reimagine the story of Peter Pan with twelve rural nursing homes across Kentucky. And so began the I Won't Grow Up project.

What if creative care could be scaled?

What if we could pour it into the water of an organization so it spread through its systems to all its staff, the elders, and their families?

What if we could transform the place people never want to go into a Neverland of wonder and imagination—of meaning and connection?

The Plan and the Team

It would be great fun to create original plays in nursing homes, but to really scale creative care, we had to make sure that what we taught and what we built could be sustainable and cost effective. It had to stick.

So Angie and I clustered the twelve nursing homes into three regions, picking homes that were close enough together that a regional artist in residence could visit them in a day without having to stay the night. That artist in residence would guide all four homes in the region toward staging the play at one "lead" site. We interviewed and selected a range of artists. Bob Martin, a theater artist with deep roots in eastern Kentucky, would take the eastern region. Andee Rudloff, a well-known muralist based in Bowling Green, would take the westernmost of our regions. And Cheyenne Mize, a nationally recognized musician based in Louisville, would lead the four homes in the central region. All three were well connected to other artists in the region who could join in the effort as we neared performance time.

We also layered in a national team of artists to provide consistency across the sites. I would serve as "lead artist" and playwright. Iega Jeff, a Chicago-based choreographer, would guide the movement. Nicole Garneau, with national experience and a home base in Kentucky, would be our production manager. And Jeff Becker, a New Orleans–based designer with a specialty in staging plays in unconventional places, would handle design. And, boy, was this going to be an unconventional setting. To make the team, each artist had to have three things: (1) deep and successful experience working with nonartists; (2) experience making highly recognized professional work; and (3) little to no ego. As with the SAIR program, I was open with folks I talked to about this work not being for everyone. Artists couldn't be married to a vision. This work demanded total flexibility and trust. The play would need to be shaped in call-and-response form so that a new person might happily join in on the last day of performance. We would need to create a path for the ambulance gurney to cut through each scene—just in case. People we grew close to over the year might die before the performance. Still, it would all be worth it.

Each of the twelve homes identified two staff members to lead the initiative: the director of quality of life and the director's assistant. The nursing home administrators all signed off on the project, and more than 75 percent of staff watched an introductory video explaining what the heck was happening. Angie and I structured the training in waves, allowing time for the staff to absorb the shift away from directing activities and toward inviting expression and building on elders' imagination and input. We would have a kick-off training, with all the lead staff and artists gathered together, followed by a series of residencies by regional and national artists. With each residency, we would deepen the exploration of the story. Eventually we would all gather again for a retreat to draft the script and then turn our heads and hearts toward creating the play itself.[3]

Unpacking the Story

Before Angie and I assembled all the players for our kick-off training, I fell down the rabbit hole of the story of Peter Pan. I had already been exploring the idea in Milwaukee in partnership with Meals on Wheels, but now I watched every movie. I read the play, the novel, the musical. I worked with a similarly obsessed graduate student to assemble a guide that broke the story into hundreds of beautiful questions that explored key themes:[4]

What do you know of the story of Peter Pan?

Can you tell it in three sentences? Three words?

Can you tell it only in movements? Can you add sounds?

What exactly is the meaning of childhood, this state that Peter clings to?

What are the sounds and the tastes? The feelings? The games?

And on the flip side, what was this thing that Peter was so afraid of?

What are the sounds and tastes and feelings of adulthood?

The story is ripe with themes of care, home, and, of course, flying. In the novel, the children's nanny is a beloved Newfoundland dog named Nana. We would have to slip around the inappropriateness of comparing caregivers to dogs and instead focus on unconditional love.

Have you experienced unconditional love?

Have you given it?

What might it feel like?

How might you show it to someone?

When Wendy crash-lands into Neverland, the Lost Boys build a house around her. Home is such a potent theme for people trying to create a new home, likely their last, in late life, while trying to hold tight to memories of the homes that shaped who they are.

What does home mean to you?

If you could build one now, what would it be like?

Flying is what everyone remembers about the story of Peter Pan. Flying is also an enormously powerful image for people with limited mobility and would need to be central to whatever story we tell.

What does it feel like to fly?

If you could fly, where would you go?

Who would you invite to go with you?

What would you see along the way?

There are some pretty cringeworthy colonialist representations in the story, too (think Tiger Lily), which seemed to thicken as the story evolved from the stage to a novel to a classic Disney movie. Gender roles have changed drastically as well. I grimaced more than once in the course of my research. But J. M. Barrie's play was also more brilliant than I had imagined. With deft humor, Barrie depicts Peter's eternal youth as less something to admire than a condition to be pitied. Wendy is the real winner here. As alluring as Peter's bravado is, Wendy is the one whose path we want to follow. She has the adventure of a lifetime. And she returns home safely to grow up and experience giving and receiving the love that Peter could never know. The trade-off for such love—aging and mortality—is clearly worth it.

Teaching Creativity and Inviting Imagination

During the very first training workshop in Kentucky, the story's power was palpable. The whole team was gathered at the elegant Brown Theatre in downtown Louisville.[5] Directors of quality of life from each of the twelve homes were there with elders the directors had brought with them. Our team of regional and national artists joined the workshop as well. The initial training was two full days. In small groups of artists mixed with elders, caregivers, and staff, we toggled between explaining the project and art-making experiences. We painted. We sang. We wrote poems. We made wordless statues with our bodies. Using the Brown Theatre lobby, we explored how to interpret the emotional feeling of physical spaces, and then how to transform them with story. "Reading spaces" is a difficult concept for nonartists to grasp, but ultimately, this will be our most powerful tool. Children know this inherently—that beds can become boats and a bedroom a vengeful sea. But adults need reminding. A nursing home dayroom can become Cape Canaveral. Wheelchairs can become rocket ships.

It was in Iega Jeff's workshop that I felt that knowledge sink down from our minds and seep into our muscles, sinews, and souls. I had asked him to guide us through a movement exercise on flying. Iega is six feet, seven inches, and every movement he makes is a study in grace. His Chicago-based dance company is called Deeply Rooted and that is the feeling one gets in his presence: that his movements and actions are deeply connected to his history, his community, his values—to all that he is. Iega came up before the room of sixty people, seated in small groups around round tables, and simply asked them to close their eyes and breathe. I got a little nervous. One thing I know from doing this work for a long time now is that artists can seem opaque to nonartists—flaky or weird might be a more direct way to put it. Inviting people too quickly into an exercise that would be normal in a rehearsal room might alienate the more left-brained, nonartist people in the room. Or was I projecting my own apprehensions?

After breathing in silence, Iega guided us a little deeper. "We'll do the same thing, only this time, just imagine your body is starting to lift up," he said. We would all stay seated, but just imagine the very first feelings of weight shifting from heaviness to lightness. Iega slowly added music to these brief imaginings, and gradually guided us through actual flight. "Let your body lead you where it wants to go, let your arms lift, or come to a stand, whatever it wants, whatever is possible." Slowly, he was linking our thoughts, our feelings, and our movement. I stopped worrying about what the nonartists were thinking and fell into the exercise. I found myself in a pool as a kid, kicking off from the side wall and gliding into the middle of the water. I stood up slowly, imagining the gliding sensation and the peacefulness of feeling weightless. Iega had led us through such a gradual and subtle evolution of complexity that I was breathless when I cheated and opened my eyes, looked around the room, which was silent save for Iega's music. Some people stood, their arms high above them. Others had their arms gently swaying to the side. Some remained seated, their chins lifting subtly upward. Some of the elders that Signature staff brought to the workshop were in their wheelchairs, hands and fingers pointed skyward, clearly soaring. It was a room of flight.

Iega asked us to reflect. I was still cautious about asking so much of the group—to feel these enormous feelings and translate them into words. Performers are used to this. But quality of life directors? Nursing assistants? Elders? Family caregivers? I remember feeling my breath grow more shallow. "Where did you go? What did you see?" Iega asked. It was quiet for a moment. Then, slowly, people began to respond. They flew over family farms, describing the curve of the landscape and the joy of seeing it again as they remembered it. They flew to see grandchildren. One woman flew over the cemetery and then to heaven to see a child who had died. When people finished responding, Iega held the silence in the room for a moment, honoring the breadth of emotions, balancing the lightness of the joy with the weight of sorrow and loss. This powerful experience was in the first three weeks of the three-year project. We knew we were going to train the staff. We knew we were focusing on the Peter Pan story, and gradually building a play at three of the twelve homes. While we did not know what that play would be yet, clearly we would be doing this exercise again. And again and again.

Over the next couple of months, the staff completed TimeSlips's online training and the artists in residence visited their sites. They modeled a whole range of creative engagement techniques and started exploring the story with staff and elders. In eastern Kentucky, Bob Martin led story workshops. In the four homes clustered around Bowling Green, visual artist Andee Rudloff invited the elders to create models of their homes and paint murals together. Closer to Louisville, musician Cheyenne Mize gathered and practiced favorite childhood songs with the elders at Hodgenville's Sunrise Manor.

The National Artists Come to Visit

Sunrise Manor is an impressive place. It is new construction with two stories, multiple courtyards, loads of natural light, and wide hallways that curve into clusters of rooms rather than the more institutional "double-loaded" corridor model. In May 2018, Angie, Iega (choreographer), Jeff (designer), Nicole (production manager), and I gathered in Louisville to begin a journey across the state and spend a couple of days at each of the lead sites in the three regions. When we hit Sunrise Manor, we made our way down to the main dining room where Cheyenne was waiting for us. When we turned the corner, I was floored. There were nearly seventy people gathered in a huge circle: elders from Sunrise and some who had traveled with the lead staff from the other three nursing homes in the region. They waved and cheered as we walked in. Cheyenne was at the "noon" spot in the circle with her guitar strapped on and standing next to a flip chart. She was ready for us.

Over in the corner, just outside of the circle, I spotted the folks from the Office of the Inspector General of the State of Kentucky's Department of Health Services. They were our funders—and overseers. They were the ones who held Angie's and my hands through the twenty-seven versions of the proposal—through the conceptual jujitsu of organizing a project to bring an iterative, creative process into one of the most regulated industries in the United States, nursing homes. "What will the play be?" these folks asked during the proposal process. "That's up to the elders," we explained. "What supplies do you need and how much will they cost?" "We won't know until we know the story of the play," we explained. These are two very different ways of thinking—two different ways of being. But if this approach was to be replicable, if it was to spread to nursing homes across the country, we would need the support of people such as these agency staff. I invited them to join the circle, but they gently declined. They preferred just to watch, from the side. Even twenty years after the initial magic with the Marlboro Man, I was worried: Would it work? Would they get it?

Iega brought a chair into the middle of the circle and warmed us up with a simple breathing exercise that opens into movement. His presence awed the room. His movements seemed to draw people into them, and they climbed as he climbed, they rolled as he rolled. Then it was Cheyenne's turn. Cheyenne exudes warmth. She has a soft, hypnotic voice and a serenity about her that makes it easy to join in to whatever activity she invites you. For this big group, on this first day of our residency, with our funders watching from outside the circle, Cheyenne handed out shakers and invited people to play with them. Then she put "Whole Lotta Shakin' Goin' On" on the speakers, and the room burst into a playful silliness. I found my way between Bradley and another gentleman. Bradley has close-cropped hair, bright eyes, and a wide smile. He was exuberant—truly beaming and shaking and swaying. The other gentleman needed a little coaxing to join. But Bradley's energy was infectious, and gradually the other elder released into a few shakes and a smile—tiny, but perceptible.

Then Cheyenne shifted gears and asked all of us what it feels like to care for someone, what it means to people. The group provided a few answers. At first, I was worried that this instruction would be too abstract, but after a moment's thought, the elders jumped in:

* Loving
* A foundation
* Feeding people
* Making sure people have what they need

Cheyenne handed out simple, flat drums and asked people to pair up. Together they would care for each other as they made music, shaking their egg shakers or beating their plastic drum rim. It was a simple mirroring exercise, so common in community arts practices, and always moving. Staff and artists partnered with elders, but many elders also partnered with each other. At first the activity was just playful. One of the partners took the egg shaker and made movements that the partner could mirror. But gradually, you could feel people's generosity as they learned each other's range of movement. One partner would lead gently. The other would repeat the movement as if it were a gift back to the first. There were two older women, both in wheelchairs (nearly everyone was in wheelchairs), guiding each other—so gently and intimately—showing such great care for each other. Another woman, who couldn't speak, would make sounds during part of the song and hit her foot on the ground to the beat. For what I remember as nearly fifteen full minutes, we created a soundscape of care and tenderness in offering and repeating rhythms.

Cheyenne wrapped up the morning session by inviting us to create and sing a simple song set to a classic folk tune that everyone in the room could either recognize or easily learn: "Building a Home." We sang it several times through and created movements/gestures for the song and performed them. Cheyenne invited the group to change the lyrics by asking for their thoughts on what a community or a home should feel like:

*   Very friendly
*   Small
*   Sharing
*   Homelike
*   Loving

* Good

* Cleanliness

* Real good—real real good
  (This was Bradley's contribution.)

* Compassion

* Courageous

* Fun—a true foundation

Iega invited us to create movements for each idea, and Cheyenne guided us through replacing the song's original lyrics with ours. We sang the song multiple times through. It was truly elevating: you could feel the room swell with pride at writing the song, singing it, and doing movements that we created to it. It was ours, together. And we had cared for one another in the creation of it.

I kept watching one woman, sitting on the opposite side of the room from me, right next to Cheyenne's flip chart. She was in a vibrant teal blouse. She was quite thin and frail, pitched sharply to her side in the wheelchair. Yet her eyes and expression seemed to draw her upward. In every movement exercise she lifted her fingers to the farthest edge of her limited range of movement. She was deeply engaged, offering her full self. After Cheyenne finished, I found my way over to the woman in teal and told her that I loved watching her movements. They were beautiful in their emotion and intention. She smiled. I wasn't sure whether she believed me or thought I was laying it on thick for her. But I was genuinely moved. After a pause, she asked me if I had any literature on this project so she could read more about it. "This was challenging," she said. "They underestimate us here."

As the morning session broke up for lunch, Jeff, our designer, and Nicole, our production manager, gathered the administrators and building maintenance team for their "creative asset mapping" lunch meeting. Their goal? To understand all talents and resources in the community that we might build upon as part of the playmaking process. Who plays instruments? Which parts of the building could be used as natural gathering places? What special skills do people have? Too often people think of nursing homes as places of loss. Even the staff can think this way. Nicole, in her endearing way, set about flipping that frame and inviting people to see all their strengths and the potential in their building.

Meanwhile, I grabbed the keys to our long, awkward fifteen-person van (we nicknamed it the "Care-a-Van") and drove Angie and our funders to lunch—hoping desperately not to crash it. Thankfully, we made it to a restaurant in the next town over without incident. Also thankfully, our lunch conversation was easy and revealing. I asked the members of our group what they had noticed in the morning session and held my breath. To my relief they marveled at the depth of engagement. It was illuminating to learn that one of them had been an activity assistant and then activity director before shifting to administration and his current job at the state. His main question, he said, remained one of sustainability. Ah, yes—sustainability. It haunted any project aimed at improving care. All projects seek innovation, but how could we make sure it stayed lodged in the organization?

I explained my approach—my hope really—that sustainability comes from putting pressure in three directions. First, you engage the next generation (students and volunteers) so that this joyful and exhilarating approach just becomes normal to them. Second, you establish the incentives that convince the institutions to keep doing the work: research on improving health and reducing costs. And third, you engage and share stories with families and neighbors about the power of the work, so the larger community puts pressure on the institutions to keep up the change. Hundreds of people calling care homes and agencies to say, "Why aren't you doing this?" will drive sustainability. Education, research, and story—we were doing all three. We were engaging young people as volunteers. Our research team was assessing whether we could improve mood and reduce depression (thereby reducing costs of care). And we were inviting families and the extended community into the wonderment of the project. But it was also becoming clear that we needed to encourage staff (and elders and family) to identify the next project before this one was over so they could imagine the future even as they were taking their first steps into creative care. What would be the next story they would tackle after Peter Pan?

The afternoon session was filled with more storytelling with sound and movement. At the end of the day, I gathered staff who were completing their official training and I held a short reflection period with them. About a dozen of us gathered elbow to elbow around a conference room brimming with papers and training materials. "What did you see?" I asked. They described being surprised by the level of engagement. They saw people open up and were inspired. And they noted they were as well—open and inspired. "What was it about the facilitation that made that happen?" I asked.

There were no wrong answers.

You are patient with answers.

There were lots of ways to answer. If someone didn't have words, they could respond with sound or movement.

They created things, themselves.

It felt important.

I truly could not have said it better myself.

Shaping the Script

The structure that Angie and I put together for the project was like a series of waves that intensified over time. The initial training was followed by a period for the staff's own creative self-discovery, and then a series of residencies with artist visits, which would eventually lead to the shaping of a script for the performances at the three lead homes. With each visit with the arts team, both the process and the ideas for the play became clearer. Somewhere in the midst of the first residency, Angie and I realized that people at Signature HealthCARE's corporate office needed a better understanding of what was happening in the field. They were confused. "You're performing Peter Pan? How cute!" tended to be the sentiment. The project was so much deeper than that. Still, it was hard to explain. We needed to find a way to bring them into the process. So we decided to hold the two-day devising retreat at Signature's corporate headquarters itself.

Devising is really a fancy word for "making it up." Our goal for the two-day devising retreat as we gathered in September 2018 was to review all the incredible creative responses that were pouring out of the twelve nursing homes and to see how we might build a story out of it. Which ideas and themes were resonating most? What kind of story might those ideas and themes tell? By the end of the retreat, I was to miraculously come up with a loose script for the three performing sites—no pressure!

Signature HealthCARE's corporate headquarters is in a suburban office park just east of Louisville. On the day of the retreat, the training room was filled with display tables, one from each of the twelve homes, telling the story of the workshops they had done. After the May residency, the artistic team had sent out a list of creative challenges, and both the range and depth of the responses were remarkable. We asked the quality-of-life directors to invite residents to explore the symbolism of the Crocodile in *Peter Pan*. Residents of one home made a giant drawing of a crocodile and invited the children from the summer camp and their elders to write their fears inside its belly. They hung it up in a prominent hallway. Residents of another home made dozens of little crocodiles out of clothespins. The tiny crocodiles clamped their mouths shut on a piece of paper on which people had written their fears. There were original songs, and letters from Wendy to Peter, and fairy houses—lots and lots of fairy houses. For one of our creative challenge requests, we had asked the staff to work with elders to "enchant" several areas of their home. Some of the enchanted areas should be in the open. And some, we said, should be hidden—in drawers or out-of-the-way places—to be discovered like a secret. One of my favorite photos on the display boards was of a regular filing cabinet drawer, marked with a sign that read, "Shhh, Fairies Sleeping." In the next shot, the drawer was open and full of moss, sparkles, and a tiny house. All of this incredible creativity would eventually be folded into the play.

Overall, the devising retreat was balanced between reviewing what the homes were doing and exploring forward a bit by playing scenes from the moments of the story that the elders were finding the most resonant. Some of the folks from corporate joined us, watching as we pretended to be pirates, embodied our fears of the ticking Crocodile, and imitated the flying of fairies. Most moving was a much anticipated moment when Joe Steier, Signature's CEO, was able to join us for a few minutes. He came in the room just as we were sharing our thoughts about the power of opening ourselves and the elders to imagination. After hearing the quality-of-life directors talk about how this project is transforming the way they think about their work, Joe stood up to make a few comments. "I've always loved the story of Peter Pan," he said. "I was adopted, so in some ways I always felt like a Lost Boy. What you are doing," he told the room, "is so powerful." He pointed to some of our songwriting on flip-chart paper that we'd posted around the room. It perfectly captured the range of emotions in our work, from irreverent and silly to deeply wise, all while honoring the emotional and physical pain and loss that can present themselves in late life:

If I could tell Peter what I know now, I'd tell him
Aging's not bad.
If I could tell Peter what I know now, I'd tell him
Enjoy the moments.
About making memories, and difficult times,
Don't worry about a thing, 'cuz the bad times won't last.
And eat lots of junk food while your metabolism's fast!
If I could tell Peter what I know now, I'd tell him
I love you, don't go.

"It's exactly what we are trying to show people, to enjoy the moments, that aging doesn't have to be bad," offered Steier. Some of the quality-of-life directors had never met their CEO in person. He was fully present. He got what we were doing. He praised the work of some staff members by name. The moment packed quite an emotional wallop. Cheyenne and I made eye contact, but she was already on it, grabbing her guitar and heading up to the front of the room. As a thank-you to Joe for saying yes to this experiment of integrating the creative process and serious culture-making into twelve of his company's homes, the whole room sang him the song. I managed not to cry, but I did notice that some of the staff were tearing up. Angie pulled me aside and said simply, "I'm so happy."

The Story Takes Shape

A year into the project, we had a script at last. Built from the interests and skills of the elders and staff, the story went like this:

Wendy is on hospice care. She has been living at the nursing home for the past ten years and is beloved by everyone who works and lives there. Wendy emanates an aura of goodness and regales everyone who will listen with magical stories of pirates and fairies, of Peter, Lost Boys, and crocodiles. Although everyone is riveted by her tales, no one quite believes them. They think perhaps she read the book or saw the movie a few too many times. Regardless, the staff and residents have decided to honor Wendy's last days by re-creating the world of her stories, and they invite the audience to share in the experience with them. As audience members walk from the parking lot to the front of the home, they'll be treated to surprise scenes with pirate fights, scrappy Lost Boys, and sleeping fairies. The staff and elders explain the story to audience members and welcome them to three interactive stations. First is "Positive Thoughts," where people write a thought that can help them fly. Second is the "Crocodile" station, where audience members are invited to write their fears on canning lids, which will soon become the scales of the Crocodile. The third station is the magical "Flight School," where audience members can experience flying, guided by elders, staff, and volunteers.

From Flight School, strolling musicians lead the audience deeper into the nursing home, to a place called Wendy's Story Room. This is where Wendy holds court. The walls are covered in letters from Wendy to Peter, songs, and other artifacts. Audience members can pick up headphones and listen to recordings of elders reading the stories or singing the songs aloud. Suddenly, the Lost Boys rush through the room—"Wendy! There she is!"—and curtains suddenly open to reveal Wendy and her friend Tick Tock the Crocodile sitting on the patio together, with Tick Tock in a heavy coat adorned with all of our fears. The two of them are relaxing and reminiscing. We can hear their thoughts on the headphones, prerecorded to enable Wendy to be played by an elder without the burden of memorization. Tick Tock is sad that Wendy is dying soon, but she comforts him: "I'm just finishing growing up, Tick." He marvels that she is not afraid of him and wonders whether she is afraid of anything. "Oh, yes," she says. "I am afraid that no one believes me." Tick Tock assures her that he believes her. She raises a hand to him, and he presses his own against her palm: two hands in one prayer. "I am Wendy," she says. "I am licorice snaps. I am love. I am Neverland. I am at peace." Wendy falls asleep, and Tick Tock rises to inspire the audience to believe to help Wendy be free to fly away at last. We follow him to the dining hall, past more antics of Lost Boys and sleeping fairies. When we arrive in the dining hall, we see portraits of elders from all twelve participating homes on translucent paper strung around the room. We hear an audio recording of elders, again from all twelve homes, reciting poems about their own stories: their name, a childhood game, something they are proud of, a place they love, a feeling. Poems like those the staff gathered over the past months:

I am Lorene.
I am playing school.
I am saved.
I am my old home place.
I am alright.
I am Jake.
I am making a windmill.
I am a hunter.
I am the hills.
I am fine.
I am Freddie.
I am throwing a ball.
I am a dad.
I am McKee.
I am real good.
I am Pauline.
I am wading in the creek.
I am a mother.

I am Florida, Ohio, everywhere.

I am o.k.

I am Jimmie.

I am riding my bicycle.

I am a big brother.

I am Grandpa's place.

I am restless.

I am Mary.

I am playing on the hill.

I am God's child.

I am here with you.

I am loving.

There is a chorus of elders in wheelchairs gathered in a circle in the main room. As the audio recording fades, each one, simply and clearly, offers his or her name to the Crocodile. "I am . . ." Then in unison they say, "We are Wendy." Turning to the audience, which is gathered around the circle, they ask, "Will you believe?" And slowly each elder raises a hand to the audience. Here is a moment of trust. The story teaches audience members how to show their belief when the Crocodile matches Wendy's hand in the previous scene. Will they step forward to meet the hands of the elders? Will the audience believe? We hope they do, but we build in a backup plan just in case, with the staff, volunteers, and other elders stepping in.

When all hands are paired, we hear the sweet sounds of Frank Sinatra singing "Fly Me to the Moon." The elders and their care partners begin the "Flying Dance," with fingers, heads, hands, arms, and full bodies soaring with the power of belief. One of the elders crows like a rooster, signaling the arrival of Peter. The Crocodile speaks to his friend: "You're free, Wendy! They believe! You can fly now." And together the elders and Crocodile bid her farewell.

The scene transitions as strolling musicians beckon us to follow them back through the home and out under the drive-through awning. Along the way, we notice that the sleeping fairies are now awake. Bubbles come out of offices. Little enchantments are visible everywhere. We gather around, and the musicians and elders lead us through a rousing, choreographed version of "I'll Fly Away." As we finish, an old pickup truck pulls up to the building and two characters get out. They are the characters from the play that the nursing home has decided will be the subject of their next play project. The staff welcome them, start the admission process, and invite the audience to help them tell the next story. "If you're not already, volunteer, visit, join us as we start our next project!"

What if the cultural programming in a care home was so interesting that families and neighbors wanted to participate alongside the elders?

Engaging Neighbors

The artists ventured back for another residency in mid-November, just as the rains were forecast to turn to ice. This time, thankfully, we rented a shiny, new black sport utility vehicle to carry the team of artists across the state. We nicknamed the car "The Boss," because it made us look like we were in the Secret Service. So we thought we'd be okay. But the native Kentuckians on our team knew that even if our car could brave the roads, ice shuts everything down. "This isn't Milwaukee, Anne," said Angie. "We don't have all those salt trucks down here." We were scheduled to be at Morgantown's nursing home that day, and word had it that Andee, the incredibly energetic artist in residence for the site, had worked with staff to arrange for a hundred volunteers to be there for a special morning activity and then for many of them to stay for our afternoon workshops. They were neighbors, members of the Butler County Artists Guild, and members of the area high school Reserve Officer Training Corps (ROTC) group. We had hoped to draw new volunteers to the sites, but this response was beyond any of our expectations—way beyond.

Nicole, our production manager, hopped on the phone. The biggest group of volunteers were scheduled for 9 a.m., so they would be able to get home before the storm. We shifted our plans to arrive around noon and condense our visit to let staff and the volunteers who were able to stay to join us and still leave early. When we finally pulled into Morgantown and walked into the great room, there was a magical buzz. Staff and elders were wearing yellow, translucent wings. Some were sporting tutus. All along the long counter of the reception area and nurses' station at the back of the room were teacups and saucers. The teacups were tipped on their sides and filled with moss, flowers, and a good bit of glitter. The group had created dozens upon dozens of fairy gardens.

Our team had two goals that week on our visits to the three "lead" homes. First, we had to find the route that the play would travel through the care home. Second, Iega needed to explore the culminating flying scene with the staff and elders. He had a general choreography that had developed over the week, but each group would need to make it uniquely their own. Jeff, the designer; Bobby, the director; Andee, the site's artist in residence; and I headed off to map the route, and Iega and Nicole worked with staff to assemble the thirty-some elders gathered in the great room who would learn to fly. Iega set up his portable speaker, filling the room with Frank Sinatra's "Fly Me to the Moon." Things must have gone well. When I circled back, the room was giddy with energy. In the final move of the choreography, the care partners embraced the elders in the chairs before them. I noticed a middle-aged gentleman watching the moment from the side of the room. He looked overwhelmed, uncertain how to process what he was seeing. He caught my eye and walked over to me.

"Are you with this group?" he asked.

"I'm the lead artist, yes," I said, hoping that was a good thing in his eyes.

"I'm the police chief of this town," he told me. "My office is next door, but I haven't been in this building since I was twelve." It turned out that his grandfather had died in this nursing home, and afterward the chief had wanted to stay far, far away. But today had changed his mind. "I never imagined this would be possible," he said. "Wanting to be here—actually enjoying being here." He wanted to know how he could help, how he could be involved. I told Angie about our conversation. "Oh, I can help him figure out how to help!" she said, and she made a beeline over to him. They talked for thirty minutes.

Happy Tears—and Sad Ones, Too

During that November residency, Jeff and I were lost in wonder as we walked the route at Lee County Rehabilitation Center, the lead site in the eastern region. The "Belief" scene would happen in the main dining hall. Then the offices all along the hallway to the front of the home could be transformed with bubble machines, wings, and all other manner of fairy mischief. We were giddy about the story. The more we told it, the more powerful it felt. It resonated with the staff. The elders understood it deeply. It built on all their input and strengths. As Jeff and I walked into the lobby, we were imagining bubble machines and fairies, now awake with the power of belief. Across the lobby from us was a couple, a man and a woman in their sixties, holding each other as she wept. Enormous, exhausting, heaving sobs.

Jeff and I shared a moment of quiet, reminded of what Iega taught us in that very first workshop: that we must hold space for both loss and magic—for growth and wonder and sorrow and loss. All of that was part of this Neverland—part of the beauty and wisdom that comes with growing up. More than any other, it is this moment that is the essence of creative care.

And we did hold that space. On opening day in Morgantown, the elders' faces were wide with wonder. The staff and artists kept a list of "victories" that grew longer and longer with each performance. Shirley hadn't been out of her room since October (it was March). She was now playing the Queen of the Fairies. Renia, who played Wendy, was overwhelmed when her daughter embraced her after her big scene with the Crocodile. Charles never participated in activities and spent much of the time swearing at staff. In the last performance in Morgantown, he joined the dance chorus, and with a jaunty hat as a costume, danced in his chair to "Fly Me to the Moon," embracing his care partner in the finale. Mary hadn't been out of her room for months either, as she adjusted to an amputation. She was at every performance, costumed as a fairy, emanating joy. Gaylen's sister said she hadn't seen him this happy in years. The gurney came through several rehearsals. And dear Dimple, who had participated nearly every day, passed away just weeks after the performance. The rehearsals and performances of *Wendy's Neverland* were full of happy tears and sad ones too.

After the performances, after Ruth cried her happy tears on opening day in Morgantown, and after so many people came out of their rooms for the first time to be part of the magic-making, I returned to the question that our funders had asked so pointedly: What about sustainability? It was hard for me to believe that the magic could fade. Interviews and case studies drawn from the staff showed that they "got it" in the deepest way possible. We planned to have photos of the performance framed and hung in each of the lead sites to help lock the feelings and stories of the experience into the memory of the building itself. We had the staff of each nursing home pick the story they wanted to tell the following year. People at one of the nonlead sites insisted on doing their own performance of *Wendy's Neverland*, so we adjusted the script so it wasn't quite so dependent on Jeff's innovative set design. Once all twelve sites selected the next story they wanted to tell, we would help them identify possible themes and draft questions to start the process over again. The sites had significantly expanded their volunteer base and formed relationships with local and regional artists. The sites had all the tools to make it happen again and again.

But I was also haunted by another question: Did sustainability for an arts-based program mean it didn't merit any further investment? These elders were loaded with prescriptions. So many pills. They just kept coming and coming and coming. Some of them came with black box warnings and significant side effects. Were these pills sustainable? The system didn't seem to ask whether they were worth further investment. The system just finds a way to keep paying for the pills. Were joy and meaning-making worth it? Were feeling part of something bigger and creating a legacy worth it? Was ending soul-crushing isolation worth it? Were engaging staff and volunteers and transforming the way people saw both the elders and the care home worth the ongoing investment of collaborating with artists and not just relying on staff to deliver this program? We could give the staff all of our tools and charts and processes. But elders and staff alike would come and go, and come and go. It seems we need to find a way to prescribe meaning and joy.[6] And now, thanks to Shirley and Ruth, Angie and Iega, and every single person who contributed to that bold dream in Kentucky, we know exactly how to deliver it. We could bring it to every nursing home. We could bring it to every person who received Meals on Wheels. To all those who needed it, whether living in their own apartments or at a nursing home.

Facing the Future

In May 2016, a Milwaukee couple were found by a longtime friend and neighbor, sitting in their van, bottles of sedative on the car floor and the ashy remains of a portable grill in the back. A note—"Danger, Carbon Monoxide Gas"—was taped thoughtfully to the front window. The couple were just seventy-one and seventy-two. The night before, she had forgotten his name, again. A typed note on the kitchen counter said, "I am sorry to leave like this but the rules say I cannot tell you, Virginia and I are terminating."

I read about it in the paper and immediately emailed my friend, who led the local chapter of the Alzheimer's Association. We were scheduled to meet for lunch that day. Could he still come? He said yes. So we met up at one of Milwaukee's best Vietnamese buffets, settling in silently, plates aswirl with noodles.

"I'm so sorry," I said.

How does a person hold space for this level of despair?

He let out a breath. "It's been a rough week. I've been trying to see if they ever reached out to us. If they reached out to anyone."

"But what you're doing sounds exciting," he continued. I had originally asked him to lunch to brainstorm about my project to train fifty nursing homes across the state of Wisconsin to infuse creative engagement into their care systems—from everyday moments to planned activities. It was an incredible opportunity to bring the power of creativity into the lives of so many people. Over the years I'd watched again and again as imagination and creative expression dissolved the knot of anguish, loss, and grief with a shared smile, a song, a poetic turn of phrase that took your breath away.

But in the face of the "Danger, Carbon Monoxide Gas" sign, I felt like I was shooting a squirt gun at a forest fire—or a charcoal grill.

Was this the limit for creative care—where the possibility of hope is sealed off like the windows of that van?

By the end of lunch, my notepad was full. My friend and I hatched a plan to invite museums around the state to provide prompts for creative projects—little inspirations from their collections that could spark creative connections among elders and family, volunteers, and care staff.

We would seek out stories of the power of those creative connections and share them across the whole state in partnership with Wisconsin Public Radio. We sketched out phase two—when we would train more nursing homes—pouring the creative engagement approach into multiple systems in the hope that the community itself would become part of the support team and dull, perhaps, the sharpest edges of that despair.

Our plates were empty. My friend sighed, readying himself to head back to the office. The weight of the week's news rolled back over him.

"We're lucky to have you at the helm," I told him.

"Let's talk again," he said, trying to smile. "What you're doing is what gives people hope."

Creative care does give hope. Every story in this book, and the countless stories of the more than eight hundred TimeSlips facilitators across the world, all stand as testimony to that hope— the moments when people feel connected, when creative flow suspends the pain of loss. The work of creative care is the work of bringing meaning to suffering—through play and connection, through expression, through legacy. Through belonging. Through awe.

Finding a way to fund and support this work to make it sustainable is one key step forward. As the world moves toward the tripling of global rates of dementia, and we see dramatic increases in rates of loneliness and isolation among older adults, this work will certainly not be the only change we need—especially in the United States, which has no real long-term-care policy and where caregivers often go without basic health care themselves or even a living wage.

Meeting the demands of this new terrain needs the work of activists like Ai-jen Poo and organizations like Caring Across Generations and the National Domestic Workers Association, which are pushing back against stereotypes of care and advocating for fair wages and working conditions. If we are to change the experience of aging and disability, we must also change the way we understand and value care.

Meeting these demands needs the work of scholars like Arthur Kleinman and Eva Feder Kittay, whose careful thought, inspiring scholarship, and lived experience might well bring us to an integrated definition of care, which views care as reciprocal and a high point of human development.

Meeting these demands needs the work of writers, policy makers, and community organizers who are helping rethink Western concepts of death and dying. No one should be reading about a loving couple in their seventies resorting to carbon monoxide. Instead we should be reading more about the global Death Cafe movement, informal gatherings designed to increase awareness of death in order to "make the most of our (finite) lives." Or Respecting Choices, which brings an evidence-based approach in end-of-life planning to our health system.[1]

Meeting these demands needs the continuing work of Marc Freedman and his teams at Encore.org and Gen2Gen, and Donna Butts and Generations United, all working to systematically dismantle the outdated structures separating the generations.

Meeting these demands needs the exciting work happening in countries with national health systems like the United Kingdom, Australia, and Canada, which are shaping social prescription programs to open both information and funding streams between clinicians and cultural organizations. Our fractured and crisis-oriented health-care system in the United States will make social prescribing models challenging. But I have hope that eventually insurance companies will recognize the preventative impact of the arts and offer creative programming in the same way that they now offer programs like "Silver Sneakers" (subsidized gym memberships for older adults).

Meeting these demands will need the vision and talents of researchers who are starting to figure out ways to measure the complexity of generative creative relationships. Because the impact of the arts is relational, it can be messy to measure. Double-blind, randomized control studies that have been called the "gold standard" in research will not always work to best capture the benefits of arts programming in care settings.

Meeting these demands will need the strength and open hearts of family and friends caring for elders experiencing frailty, loneliness, or dementia: strength to push beyond the grief over changes they see in people, and open hearts to help invite and reveal who the person is now.

I will need my mom, who is teaching me how to experience dementia, how to accept care, and how to laugh and live even as she breathes in loss and fear.

I will need my children, who I know intuitively understand what I struggle so hard here to explain. After my mother, Sally Louise Cantwell Basting, received her official diagnosis, I wrote a letter to my sons. My boys, now seventeen and fourteen, have grown up knowing my work with elders. And they know my love of infusing creativity into our everyday lives. We still talk about the story we told walking through the woods at camp one summer. Its edges are hazy, but it involved two boys who discover a locked wooden chest in the woods, and a librarian and a secret map. We remember that we loved it. And shaped it with every step we took through the woods ourselves. When they complained that, as a Jewish family, they didn't get to celebrate Easter, we made up our own holiday called Sweet Day, complete with colors and rituals and lots and lots of candy. I hoped my letter would connect the dots for them. Between the conversations they undoubtedly overheard, my work, and our family's playful spirit, I hoped the letter would prepare them for what was to come. Perhaps I hoped the letter would do the same for me. I leave you with it here, as an accumulation of my hope and the possibility of Creative Care.

Dear Ben and Will,

You know how we've been talking about Grandma having some memory trouble? For a year it's been noticeable on the edges of our time with her. She forgot that you were meeting her at the cabin and left before you got there. She stopped making cookies (although she buys them for you!). She'll say, "What are we doing?" asking us for reminders of when and where things are happening. Grandpa has been writing everything in a little calendar by the cookie jar, which has helped a lot.

Her memory problems have not affected who she is. She's feisty. She loves to read. She loves watching the birds at the cabin. She loves when you visit and smile at her with your full being and give her your big hugs. She loves going to camp and hearing all the stories of your adventures on the trail. She loves walking down to the river and sitting on the dock there. And sitting on the dock on the lake too, watching you swim or watching the loons. She loves playing golf and playing with you guys, even though you are pretty bad, no matter how far you can hit the ball. She loves how much you love to drive the golf cart. She loves you.

Well, this week Grandma went in for a long day of testing at the neurologist's office. And he changed the diagnosis from mild cognitive impairment to what they now call "major neurocognitive disorder: probable Alzheimer's."

What does that mean?

It means that now we know that Grandma's memory changes are going to get worse. There was a chance with the mild cognitive impairment diagnosis that her memory would stay the same. But this means it won't. We'll notice more changes over time. She might get confused, worried, even scared. Imagine suddenly looking around and not knowing where you are or why you are there? That's scary. That's what can happen when the brain goes through these changes. It can take a long time, or it can happen kind of quickly—there's no telling.

It means she will love us, but sometimes she might not know it right away. It means we need to exude love for her so she can really feel it.

It means that even though it might be a little scary sometimes to see her confused, we should keep calm and exude love for her. That will calm her and us at the same time.

It means we have to get strong and not let the disease or other people interrupt our love for her.

It means that at some point, if we are out at a restaurant or at camp or anywhere really, people might feel awkward around her because they don't know what Alzheimer's is, or because they are scared of it. It means that we just exude love and acceptance and model that for them. "It's just Grandma. Relax everyone . . ." By treating her normally, others will learn to treat her normally too. It means that if anyone treats her poorly or ignores her, we gently correct them to help them better understand what Alzheimer's is. After all, fifteen million people are going to have this in ten years. They better get ready.

Some helpful one-liners:

"It's just Alzheimer's. It's not catchy."

"Let me introduce you—this is my Grandmother and I love her."

"If you ask ten people in this room if they know someone with Alzheimer's, chances are they will all say yes."

Ben, remember when a kid on your soccer team made a snide comment about Jews? And you asked if you could wear a yarmulke to practice the next week to show him you were proud to be Jewish? Feel free to have that same feisty attitude about this. You inherited that from Grandma.

Grandma is an awesome person. You have lots of great stories about her, and we can share those with her. And there's still things you don't know about Grandma that you can discover by talking with her about her growing-up times.

We love her—and she'll need our love all through this experience, all the way through to the end, because this is likely what she'll die of eventually.

Let's talk with her. Let's play with her. Let's smile at her with our full being. Let's hug her. Let's let her know in all the ways we can, that love is stronger than fear and confusion. We'll all be afraid and confused at times. Dying is a really trippy concept for humans to wrap their minds around. It's scary and profound all at the same time. We will all grow a lot by this experience. The trick is not to let death sneak in earlier than it needs to by letting our fears cut us off from each other. She will want to know, now and later, too, that you are living and loving your own lives too. Soccer, school, music, friends, camp—all of it.

It means that this might get hard for Grandpa, and Aunt Ellen, Uncle Tom, and me, too. We will be sad, because Grandma is a really special person. She was and is a really, really good mom, and I actually learned a lot about being a mom from her. If you think about things you like about me, chances are I actually got that from Grandma. Grandpa is going to miss their old times—they traveled all over the world and ran marathons and did amazing backpacking and canoe trips together. So sometimes, if you see us being sad, it's okay. It's like a wave that moves through you now and then.

But again, the trick is not to let fear or sadness keep us from loving each other. Alzheimer's might well move slowly. But even if it moves quickly, we can laugh and play and invite her into the moment with us. We can live and love and play all the way to the end. Together, with Grandma, we'll learn about how to be incredible human beings.

Love you guys. Life's an adventure.

ACKNOWLEDGMENTS

A Bit on the Writing Process and Boundless Gratitude

Some of the stories I tell here are well over thirty years old. I relay them as best I can, but inevitably the dialogue is as close an approximation as I can make it. In cases where I have written or recorded notes (my experiences with Bill, Fran, and Jim; video of TimeSlips sessions; student field notes; and my own field notes from various projects), I was able to cite dialogue or comments verbatim.

There are so many people who have accompanied and inspired me on my journey through this work over the past thirty years that this section risked being longer than the book itself. So I will resort to a sampling and beg forgiveness.

Thank you to my parents for their generosity and bravery in letting me share their story here. In the beginning, I wrote them questions and they responded by email. They talked with me by speakerphone, processing everything that was happening through the diagnosis and various decisions. Dad mailed me copies of all the diagnostic papers. He read every chapter through all various drafts and offered feedback. I read chapters aloud to Mom as well. I wanted to make sure, as best I could, that my memories hadn't strayed too far into imagination and that she was okay with my sharing stories of her experiences. She was, and I'm grateful.

I thank Kathleen Woodward in every book I write. Without her blazing the trail with her research in aging and the humanities, and without the many, many letters of support and connections to people and opportunities she offered, none of my work would be possible.

I stepped into the field of arts and aging as it was just starting to emerge, with the work of people like the late Gene Cohen and his Center for Aging, Health and Humanities; Arthur Strimling and his team at Roots & Branches Theater; Susan Perlstein and the work of Elders Share the Arts; Stewart Kandell and Stagebridge; Pam Schweitzer and the Intergenerational Reminiscence Center; and Ann McDonough and the Senior Theatre Festival at the University of Nevada, Las Vegas.

I've grown up in the field alongside generous peers, discovering each new footstep together: Gary Glazner and the Alzheimer's Poetry Project; John Zeisel of I'm Still Here; David Leventhal and the Mark Morris Dance for PD (Parkinson's disease) program; Maria Genne and Kairos Alive; Judith Kate Friedman and Songwriting Works; Francesca Rosenberg and Carrie McGee at the Museum for Modern Art; Elizabeth Lokon and Opening Minds Through Art; Gay Hanna and then Jenni Smith Peers at the National Center for Creative Aging; Maura O'Malley and Ed Friedman of Lifetime Arts; and Dominic Campbell with Creative Aging International.

Now of course, there are many more programs designed to bring creative expression and engagement to late life, from museum programs to those embedded in libraries and senior centers. I'm proud of what we've built with TimeSlips and am incredibly thankful to the sponsors, board members, and staff who have believed in us all these years. TimeSlips has grown into an organization that believes deeply in wonder and awe and invites everyone in its orbit to let their imaginations soar. We believe firmly that creativity is innate and that the world is a better place when artists, elders, and caregivers cocreate.

My creative work is never done alone. The whole team at Sojourn Theatre waded into multiple adventures with me, especially Michael Rohd, Maureen Towey, James Hart, Rebecca Martinez, Shannon Scrofano, Nik Zaleski, and Jake Cohen, who poured their full selves into Penelope. Maureen, Shannon, Rebecca, and James continued on through into the Islands of Milwaukee and the Crossings. Dick Blau, Beth Thielen, Gülgün Kayim, Christopher Bayes, and Ellis Neder helped me early on to discover and harness the visual and theatrical power of TimeSlips stories. The I Won't Grow Up team was one of the most supportive ensembles I've ever worked with, deeply engaging with elders and staff while making truly beautiful theater. Bob Martin, Jeff Becker, Iega Jeff, Nicole Garneau, Clare Hagan, Cheyenne Mize, and Andee Rudloff were just a few members of this remarkable team. Thank you.

I am enormously grateful to my older friends who accepted me into their sphere and helped me understand what my own life experience couldn't yet imagine: Rocille McConnell, Rusty and Sharon Tym, Joyce Heinrich, and so very many others.

The TimeSlips team was incredibly good at protecting my writing days to ensure I had the time and emotional space to get this done; special thanks to Kate Britton and Angela Fingard.

My friend Toby Barlow helped me release my voice from its academic casing by texting me names of poets to read. Toby guided me to my agent, Stephanie Cabot, who helped me shape my unruly thoughts and guided me to my editor at HarperOne, Mickey Maudlin. Mickey found the gentlest of ways to get me to rethink a chapter. He and Judith Curr saw the larger potential for this work well before I could. Thank you.

In addition to my parents, I had many generous (and thankfully very honest) readers of these stories as the book evolved: Dr. Abhilash Desai, Dr. Susan McFadden, Kathryn Washington, Dan Kuhn, Marianne Lubar, Harriet Barlow, Elaine Maly, Robert Martin, Phyllis Brostoff, Angie McAllister, John McFadden, Jason Pushkar, Anny Pycha, Aims McGuinness, and Jennifer Jordan.

I'm thankful for my family's dark humor, practicality, and openness to love and frailty: Ellen and Seth Dizard, Tom Basting, and Becca Arons. My husband, Brad, has lived this work with me for twenty-five years, listened to every word of it read aloud, and offered the sometimes devastating but always apt "Have you thought of . . . ?" My boys, Ben and Will, open their hearts and minds and never think my work is strange. Thank you, boys.

NOTES

Chapter 3: When Opposites Come Together

1. It's important to note that Bohm views human creativity as part of the larger creative forces at work in the universe.

2. Hennessey and Amabile, "Creativity." *Annual Review of Psychology* 6 (1) (2010), 572.

3. James Kaufman and Ronald Beghetto add "mini C" (creativity as expressed in learning) and "pro C" (personal creativity expressed by professionals that might not be recognized by a larger public); J. Kaufman and R. Beghetto, "Beyond Big and Little: The Four C Model of Creativity," *Review of General Psychology* 13(1) (March 2009) https://doi.org/10.1037/a0013688, accessed November 8, 2018.

4. D. W. Winnicott, *Playing and Reality* (New York: Routledge, 1971), 53.

5. Aagje Swinnen and Kate de Medeiros explore the use of play in TimeSlips and the Alzheimer's Poetry Project, noting that it has been underexplored as a benefit for people with dementia and adults in general; A. Swinnen and K. de Medeiros, "'Play' and People Living with Dementia: A Humanities-based Inquiry of TimeSlips and the Alzheimer's Poetry Project," *Gerontologist* 58(2)(2018), 261–69.

6. A. Maslow, "A theory of Human Motivation." *Psychological Review* 50(4)(1943), 370–96.

7. V. Frankl, *Man's Search for Meaning: An Introduction to Logotherapy* (Fourth ed.). (Boston: Beacon Press, 1992).

8. R. J. Lifton, *The Broken Connection* (New York: Simon & Schuster, 1979); R. J. Lifton, *Witness to an Extreme Century: A Memoir* (New York: Free Press, 2011).

9. M. Csikszentmihalyi, *Flow: The Psychology of Optimal Experience* (New York: Harper & Row, 1990); M. Csikszentmihalyi, *Creativity: Flow and the Psychology of Discovery and Invention* (New York: HarperCollins, 1996).

10. You can read more about the Penelope project in chapter 10 and in the book *The Penelope Project: An Arts-Based Odyssey to Change Elder Care*, ed. Anne Basting, Ellie Rose, and Maureen Towey (Iowa City: University of Iowa Press, 2016).

11. G. Cohen, *The Creative Age: Awakening Human Potential in the Second Half of Life* (First ed.). (New York: Avon Books, 2000), 14.

12. Cohen and his wife, art therapist Wendy Miller, tested this hypothesis quite intensely as Cohen succumbed to metastic prostate cancer, writing a book together

that is unashamed of living and growing through the grip of grief and loss. W. Miller, Gene D. Cohen, and Teresa Barker, *Sky Above Clouds: Finding Our Way Through Creativity, Aging, and Illness* (New York: Oxford University Press, 2016).

13. Lene Tanggaard in *Rethinking Creativity: Contributions from Social and Cultural Psychology*, eds. Alex Gillespie and Jaan Valsiner, (New York: Routledge, 2014).

14. G. Cohen, *The Creative Age: Awakening Human Potential in the Second Half of Life* (First ed.). (New York: Avon Books, 2000), 171.

15. Daniel Engster, for example, in his effort to imagine a political theory of care in a just society, sees care as focused on our physical needs; D. Engster, *Justice, Care, and the Welfare State*, First ed. (Oxford, UK: Oxford University Press, 2015). He understands care to be "a practice that includes everything we do to help individuals to meet their vital biological needs, develop or maintain their basic capabilities, and avoid or alleviate unnecessary or unwanted pain and suffering, so that they can survive, develop, and function in society" (28). Yet simply meeting physical or biological needs may keep us alive but in emotional anguish from feeling lonely or without purpose. Others push for a broader definition, one that captures small supportive acts that enable a person and the context in which the person lives to flourish. Joan Tronto sees care as activities "that include everything we do to maintain, contain, and repair our worlds so that we can live in it as well as possible. That world includes our bodies, ourselves, and our environment"; J. Tronto, *Moral Boundaries: A Political Argument for an Ethic of Care* (New York: Routledge, 1994).

16. A. Kleinman, "Care: In Search of a Health Agenda," *Lancet* 386(9990) July 18, 2015, 240–41.

17. Sheung-Tak Cheng, Emily P. M. Mak, Rosanna W. L. Lau, Natalie S. S. Ng, and Linda C. W. Lam, "Voices of Alzheimer Caregivers on Positive Aspects of Caregiving," *Gerontologist* 56(3)(June, 2016), 451–60, https://doi.org/10.1093/geront/gnu118; D. S. F. Yu, S. T. Cheng, and J. Wang, "Unravelling Positive Aspects of Caregiving in Dementia: An Integrative Review of Research Literature," *International Journal of Nursing Studies* 79(2018), 1–26.

18. E. Kittay, "Caring for the Long Haul: Long-term Care Needs and the (Moral) Failure to Acknowledge Them," *IJFAB: International Journal of Feminist Approaches to Bioethics* 6(2)(2013), 66–88.

19. Daisy Fancourt gives a sweeping overview of thirty thousand years of history of arts and health in an all-too-brief chapter of *Arts in Health: Designing and Researching Interventions* (New York: Oxford University Press, 2017). She points to the institutionalization of medical practices in clinics, hospitals, and medical schools as the moment of greatest separation between arts and culture and healing spaces. Hospitals quickly became a place where you left your culture with your clothing, folded up in the closet, while you submitted your body for medical attention.

Chapter 5: Beautiful Questions

1. I first heard the interview between Krista Tippett and David Whyte, titled "The Conversational Nature of Reality," on April 7, 2016, but it is available in the *On Being* archives at http://onbeing.org.

2. Stan Berg's blog can be found at https://www.junebergalzheimers.com/disappearing-friends.

3. Research on loneliness I drew from O. Sagan & Eric D. Miller. *Narratives of Loneliness: Multidisciplinary Perspectives from the 21st Century* (Explorations in mental health series). (Abingdon, Oxon; New York: Routledge, 2018), 13.

Chapter 6: Proof of Listening

1. A. Gawande, "Hellhole," *The New Yorker* 85(7)(2009), 36.

2. J. Stauffer, *Ethical Loneliness: The Injustice of Not Being Heard* (New York: Columbia University Press, 2015).

3. Learn more about Remen's work on generous listening in her video, which can be found at http://www.rachelremen.com/generous-listening/.

Chapter 7: Connecting to the Larger World

1. S. Wolf and John Koethe, *Meaning in Life and Why It Matters*. University Center for Human Values series. (Princeton: Princeton University Press, 2010.)

2. American Occupational Therapy Association, in a section called "What is Occupational Therapy?" https://www.aota.org/Conference-Events/OTMonth/what-is-OT.aspx.

3. M. Ikiugu, "Meaningful and Psychologically Rewarding Occupations: Characteristics and Implications for Occupational Therapy Practice," *Occupational Therapy in Mental Health* 35(1)(2019), 40–58.

4. Viktor Frankl, *Man's Search for Meaning: An Introduction to Logotherapy* (Third ed.). (New York: Simon & Schuster, 1984), 115.

Chapter 8: Opening Yourself to Wonder

1. N. Bell, Renwick Gallery, organizer, host institution, and Smithsonian American Art Museum, organizer, issuing body. *Wonder*. Washington, DC; London: Renwick Gallery of the Smithsonian American Art Museum; in association with D Giles Limited (2015), page 11.

2. You can find the story of Liz and her aunt and uncle in Liz Lerman's book *Hiking the Horizontal: Field Notes from a Choreographer* (Middletown, CT: Wesleyan University Press, 2014).

Chapter 9: All of the Above—Cultivating Awe in Our Lives

1. J. E. Stellar, N. John-Henderson, C. L. Anderson, A. M. Gordon, G. D. McNeil, and D. J. Keltner, "Positive Affect and Markers of Inflammation: Discrete Positive Emotions Predict Lower Levels of Inflammatory Cytokines," *Emotion* 15(2) (2015), 129–133, https://doi.org/10.1037/emo0000033.

2. M. Rudd, K. Vohs, and J. Aaker, "Awe Expands People's Perception of Time, Alters Decision Making, and Enhances Well-being," *Psychological Science* 23(10) (2012), 1130–36.

3. P. Piff, P. Dietze, M. Feinberg, D. Stancato, D. Keltner, and K. Kawakami, "Awe, the Small Self, and Prosocial Behavior," *Journal of Personality and Social Psychology* 108(6)(2015), 883–99.

4. For a synopsis of the emerging science behind the study of awe, look to "The Science of Awe" (2018), a white paper written by Summer Allen, PhD, at the Greater Good Science Center, with support from the John Templeton Foundation. https://ggsc.berkeley.edu/images/uploads/GGSC-JTF_White_Paper-Awe_FINAL.pdf.

Chapter 10: Penelope, the Hero Who Never Left Home

1. There are multiple studies on the impact of TimeSlips's storytelling approach. L. J. Phillips, S. A. Reid-Arndt, and Y. Pak. "Effects of a Creative Expression Intervention

on Emotions, Communication, and Quality of Life in Persons with Dementia." *Nursing Research*, 59(2010), 417–25. L. A. Bahlke, S. Pericolosi, and M. E. Lehman. "Use of TimeSlips to Improve Communication in Persons with Moderate Late-Stage Dementia." *Journal of Aging, Humanities, and the Arts, 4* (2010), 390–405. H-Y Chen, J. Li, Y-P. Wei, P. Chen, and H. Li. "Effects of TimeSlips on Cornell Scale for Depression in Dementia Scores of Senile Dementia Patients." *International Journal of Nursing Sciences, 3*(1)(2016) 35–38. T. Fritsch, J. Kwak, S. Grant, J. Lang, R. R. Montgomery and A. D. Basting. "Impact of TimeSlips, a Creative Expression Intervention Program, on Nursing Home Residents with Dementia and Their Caregivers." *Gerontologist, 49*(2009), 117–126. D. R. George and W. S. Houser. "'I'm a Storyteller!': Exploring the Benefits of TimeSlips Creative Expression Program at a Nursing Home." *American Journal of Alzheimer's Disease and Other Dementias, 29* (2014), 678–84. D. R. George, H. L. Stuckey, C. F. Dillon and M. M. Whitehead. "Impact of Participation in TimeSlips, a Creative Group-based Storytelling Program, on Medical Student Attitudes Toward Persons with Dementia: A Qualitative Study." *Gerontologist, 51*(2011), 699–713. D. R. George, H. L. Stuckey and M. M. Whitehead. "How a Creative Storytelling Intervention Can Improve Medical Student Attitude Towards Persons with Dementia: A Mixed Methods Study." *Dementia, 13*(2014), 318–29. D. R. George, C. Yang, H. L. Stuckey and M. M. Whitehead. "Evaluating an Arts-based Intervention to Improve Medical Student Attitudes Toward Persons with Dementia Using the Dementia Attitudes Scale. *Journal of the American Geriatrics Society*, 60(2012), 1583–85. A. Loizeau, Y. Kündig, and S. Oppikofer, "'Awakened Art Stories'—Rediscovering Pictures by Persons Living with Dementia Utilizing TimeSlips: A Pilot Study. *Geriatric Mental Health Care, 3*(2015), 13–20. A. A. Vigliotti, V. M. Chinchilli, and D. R. George. "Enhancing Quality of Life and Caregiver Interactions for Persons with Dementia Using TimeSlips Group Storytelling: A 6-month Longitudinal Study." *American Journal of Geriatric Psychiatry* 26(4)(2015): 507–508.

Chapter 11: From Islands to Archipelagos

1. J. Holt-Lunstad, T. Smith, M. Baker, T. Harris, and D. Stephenson. "Loneliness and Social Isolation as Risk Factors for Mortality," *Perspectives on Psychological Science* 10(2)(2015), 227–37.

Chapter 13: Let Voices Ring

1. The Unforgettables were started in 2013 out of a collaboration between New York University's Psychosocial Research and Support Program at the Center for Cognitive Neurology and the Alzheimer's Association, New York City Chapter (now Caring Kind). Dr. Mary Mittelman conducted the initial pilot research on the chorus, which is, at this writing, still going strong. The chorus rehearses for thirteen weeks, culminating in a performance of nearly twenty songs; https://med.nyu.edu/aging/research/chorus, accessed January 11, 2019.

2. The ambitious project *Love Never Forgets* was a collaboration of Giving Voice, the American Composer Forum, and the MacPhail Center for Music.

3. B. Kashyap, B. M. Stroebel, V. M. Pearsall, L. O. Erickson, and L. R. Hanson. "CHORD study: The Power of Music Through Participation in the Giving Voice Chorus," *Alzheimer's and Dementia* 14(7)(2018), P597–P598, https://doi.org/10.1016/j.jalz.2018.06.676.

4. A. Clements-Cortez. "Clinical Effects of Choral Singing for Older Adults," *Music and Medicine* 7(4)(2015), 7–12.

5. This article from the University of California, San Francisco describes the study in layperson terms: https://www.ucsf.edu/news/2018/11/412281/community-choirs-red uce-loneliness-and-increase-interest-life-older-adults, which I accessed on January 11, 2019.

   J. Johnson, A. Stewart, M. Acree, A. Napoles, J. Flatt, W. Max, and S. Gregorich. "A Community Choir Invention to Promote Well-Being Among Diverse Older Adults: Results from the Community of Voices Trial," *Journals of Gerontology: Series B*, November 9, 2018.

Chapter 14: "Wait, You *Live* Here?"

1. B. Levy, M. Slade, S. Kunkel, and S. Kasl. "Longevity Increased by Positive Self-perceptions of Aging," *Journal of Personality and Social Psychology,* 83(2)(2002), 261–70.

2. B. Levy, A. Zonderman, M. Slade, and L. Ferrucci. "Memory Shaped by Age Stereotypes Over Time," *Journals of Gerontology: Series B, 67*(4)(2012), 432–36.

3. K. Hafner. "As Population Ages, Where Are the Geriatricians?," *New York Times*, January 25, 2016. https://www.nytimes.com/2016/01/26/health/where-are-the -geriatricians.html.

4. B. Levy, P. Chung, T. Bedford, and K. Navrazhina. "Facebook as a Site for Negative Age Stereotypes," *Gerontologist* 54(2)(2014), 172–76.

5. M. Gullette. *Ending Ageism: Or How Not to Shoot Old People,* Global Perspectives on Aging (New Brunswick: Rutgers University Press, 2017).

Chapter 15: "I'm Worth Stopping For"

1. National Highway Traffic Safety Administration (NHTSA), *2017 Fatal Motor Vehicle Crashes: Overview*, Publication no. DOT-HS-812-603 (Washington, DC: US Department of Transportation, NHTSA, October, 2018). Available at https:// crashstats.nhtsa.dot.gov/Api/Public/ViewPublication/812603; https://www.ghsa .org/resources/spotlight-pedestrians18.

2. NHTSA, *Traffic Safety Facts 2015 Data—Pedestrians*, Publication no. DOT-HS-812–375 (Washington, DC: US Department of Transportation, NHTSA, February, 2017). Available at https://crashstats.nhtsa.dot.gov/Api/Public/ViewPublication/812375.

3. E. Rosén and U. Sander, "Pedestrian Fatality Risk as a Function of Car Impact Speed," *Accident Analysis and Prevention 41*(3)(2009), 536–542.

4. You can learn more about David Engwicht in Craig Raphael's profile "David Engwicht," on the People for Public Spaces website from June 28, 2009. https://www .pps.org/article/david-engwicht.

5. M. C. Caballero, "Academic Turns City into a Social Experiment," *Harvard Gazette*, March 11, 2004. https://news.harvard.edu/gazette/story/2004/03/acad emic-turns-city-into-a-social-experiment/.

6. For more on guidelines for signal length, see National Association of City Transportation Officials, "Urban Street Design Guide: Signal Cycle Lengths." https://nacto.org/publication/urban-street-design-guide/intersection-design-elements/traffic-signals/signal-cycle-lengths/. Accessed January 3, 2019.

Chapter 16: *Wendy's Neverland* or Can Creative Care Be Scaled?

1. You can learn more about the extensive evaluation of the project in *The Penelope Project: An Arts-Based Odyssey to Change Elder Care*, eds. Anne Basting, Maureen Towey, and Ellie Rose (Iowa City: University of Iowa Press, 2016).

2. Angie became a Certified Eden Instructor and has facilitated the listing of fifty-three Signature homes on the Eden Registry of the Eden Alternative, an organization that provides training for person-centered care in nursing homes.

3. The training plan for the twelve Signature nursing homes went like this: first, a two-day training institute; second, online training in the storytelling method; third, visits from the regional and national artists to demonstrate creative engagement techniques; fourth, "creative challenges" for the staff to try on their own; fifth, a two-day retreat with staff and artists to shape the play; sixth, another residency with regional and national artists to find the route of the play through the three lead sites; and finally, rehearsal and performance. Throughout, the team of artists offered creative challenges for the staff that helped guide engagement sessions with elders and volunteers.

4. I'm so thankful for the insightful work of kizzy fay, the doctoral student (and now PhD) who pored over the various texts with me and helped shape the first creativity guide for the I Won't Grow Up project.

5. We were thankful for the partnership of Kentucky's Fund for the Arts, which made the workshop in this space possible. People from this organization managed registrations, hosted a screening of the documentary about the Penelope project, and handled all logistics for this first training in Louisville.

6. Social prescribing isn't new. Early community health pioneers described writing prescriptions for food for children in Mississippi in the early 1960s and paying for the prescriptions out of their health center pharmacy budget. In the United States, references to social prescribing focus on food and housing. In the United Kingdom, Canada, and Australia, social prescribing has expanded to cover loneliness and social isolation, and has begun to refer elders to participate in meaningful creative practices to build feelings of belonging, meaning, purpose, and social support. See John Geiger, "The Unsteady March," *Perspectives in Biological Medicine* 48 (1)(2005): 1–9. I found this study cited in a recent review of social prescribing: H. A. J. Alderwick, L. M. Gottlieb, C. M. Fichtenberg, and N. E. Adler, "Social Prescribing in the U.S. and England: Emerging Interventions to Address Patients' Social Needs," *American Journal of Preventive Medicine* 54(5)(2018), 715–18.

Conclusion: Facing the Future

1. Learn more about the Death Café movement at https://deathcafe.com, and Respecting Choices at https://respectingchoices.org.